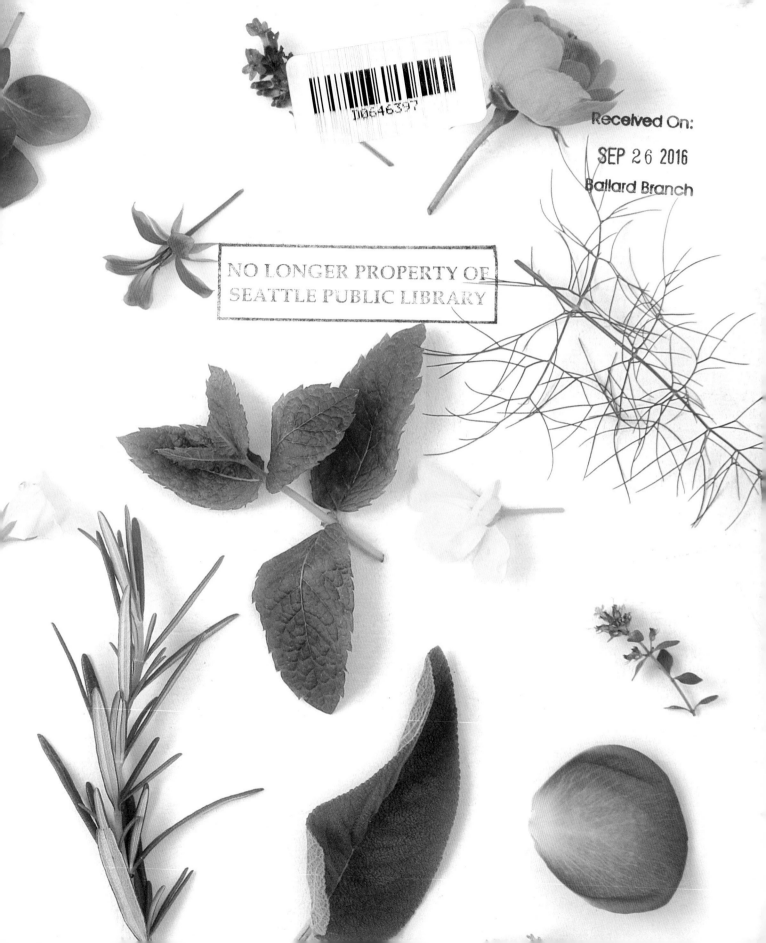

HANDMADE BEAUTY

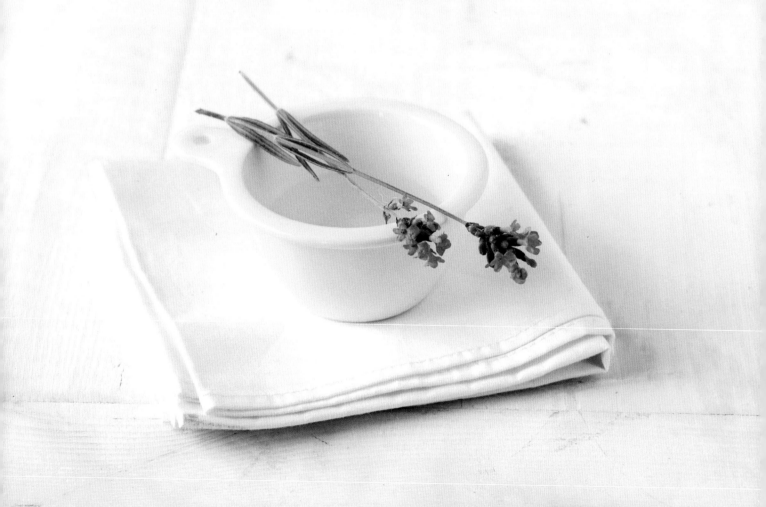

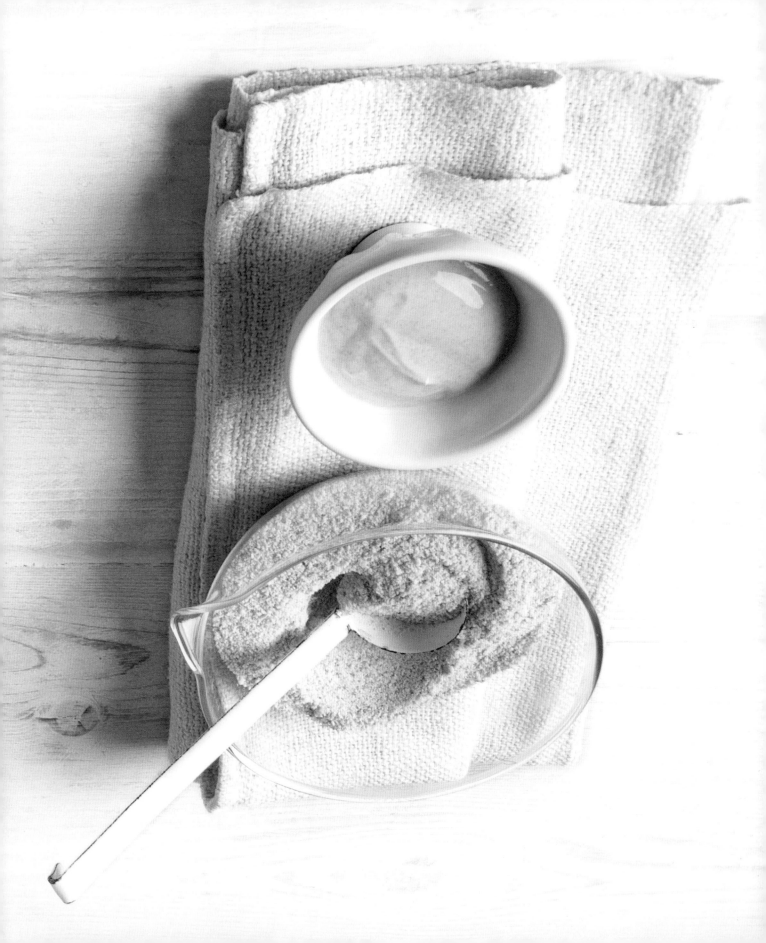

HANDMADE BEAUTY

NATURAL RECIPES FOR YOUR FACE, BODY AND HAIR

JULIETTE GOGGIN
AND ABI RIGHTON

PHOTOGRAPHY BY
AMANDA HEYWOOD

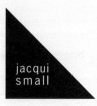

jacqui
small

First published in 2016 by
Jacqui Small LLP
74–77 White Lion Street
London N1 9PF

Publisher: Jacqui Small
Senior Commissioning Editor: Eszter Karpati
Managing Editor: Emma Heyworth-Dunn
Design and Art Direction: Rachel Cross
Editor: Claire Chandler
Photographer: Amanda Heywood
Stylist: Sophie Martell
Production: Maeve Healy

ISBN: 978 1 910254 18 9

A catalogue record for this book
is available from the British Library.

2018 2017 2016
10 9 8 7 6 5 4 3 2 1

Printed in China

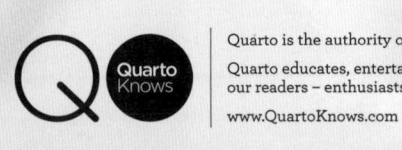

Quarto is the authority on a wide range of topics.
Quarto educates, entertains and enriches the lives of
our readers – enthusiasts and lovers of hands-on living.
www.QuartoKnows.com

CONTENTS

Introduction

No doubt about it, there's a vast array of beauty products and brands on the market today. With so much choice on offer, many of us never contemplate making our own skin- or haircare products. Or, if we do, we may be discouraged by the thought of long lists of ingredients, complicated instructions that only a chemist might follow, and expensive specialist equipment and packaging. Happily, you can forget about such concerns: this book will prove that no in-depth scientific knowledge is required, and you certainly don't have to worry about buying any test tubes. Anyone who understands the basics of cooking will find the principles of handmade skincare quite simple. In many ways, making a face cream or body lotion is similar to creating a sauce or mayonnaise – and many of us perform this task without thinking that it requires great skill.

Increasingly these days we want to know where the ingredients in our food come from, and we want to be sure that the foods we eat are as fresh as they can be, are full of taste and haven't been treated with pesticides or flown halfway across the world to reach our plates. And so now many of us like to grow our own fruit and vegetables, whether we have a generous-sized garden, an allotment or just a window box. The rise in food allergies and intolerances that are linked to stressful lifestyles also encourages us to cook more of our meals from scratch, using home-grown ingredients whenever possible.

One of our aims with this book is to make you think about handmade beauty products in the same way: a greater understanding of cosmetic ingredients and a knowledge of how beauty products are made allow us to tailor simple but effective recipes that suit our own particular skin or hair types and address specific concerns, whether that's a skin-clearing solution for an oily complexion or a soothing treatment for a dry, itchy scalp.

We have included some really quick and easy recipes that can be made in a matter of minutes, as well as more challenging projects. In total, there are 37 recipes and 10 adaptations. You will be amazed at how quickly you master the techniques involved, and also pleased to discover how inexpensive the finished products can be. It goes without saying that much of the benefit is in being able to say 'I made it myself!'

One attraction of making beauty products at home is being able to employ alternatives to the heavily perfumed, chemical-based ingredients often found in mass-produced toiletries. Our recipes feature natural ingredients (some of which you can grow in your garden or window box, or forage from the wild), and to these we add a variety of beneficial oils, butters, powders and scented essential oils, obtainable from local stores and specialist online suppliers. You are likely to want to use as many natural ingredients as possible, but it is important to remember that lots of skincare ingredients we regard as natural may be processed in some way in order to make them usable, and that not all synthetic ingredients are necessarily bad; they may be crucial to improving the performance of a product.

THE STRUCTURE OF THIS BOOK

Handmade Beauty is divided into two main parts: 'Before You Begin', which covers the types of materials you need to source, the basic equipment required and the techniques you should learn; and 'Product Recipes', which is subdivided into recipes for your face, body and hair. We know it's tempting to rush straight in and get started on the exciting recipes, but do take the time to read the first part of the book. It will help to build your confidence if you are a complete beginner to home-made beauty, and offers all-important advice not only on how to make the products safely, but also how best to store them and ensure they have the best possible shelf life.

Finding the ingredients is a large part of the fun of making your own beauty products, but you will be surprised at how many you probably already have at home. In the 'Sourcing Ingredients' section, we give you inspiration to search out some additional basics, as well as a few more enticing elements for your recipes. You can get started simply by taking stock of everyday items in your kitchen cupboard such as olive oil, sea salt and herbal teas,

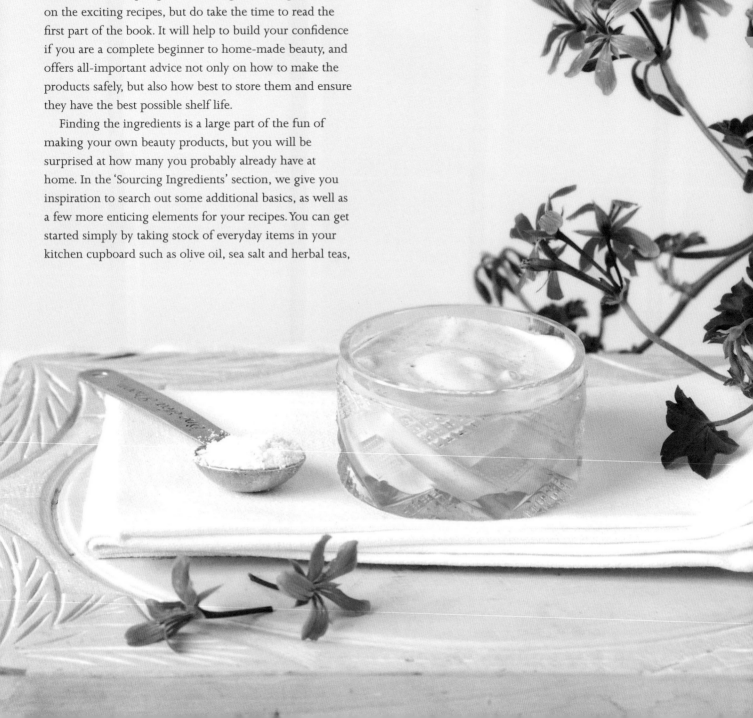

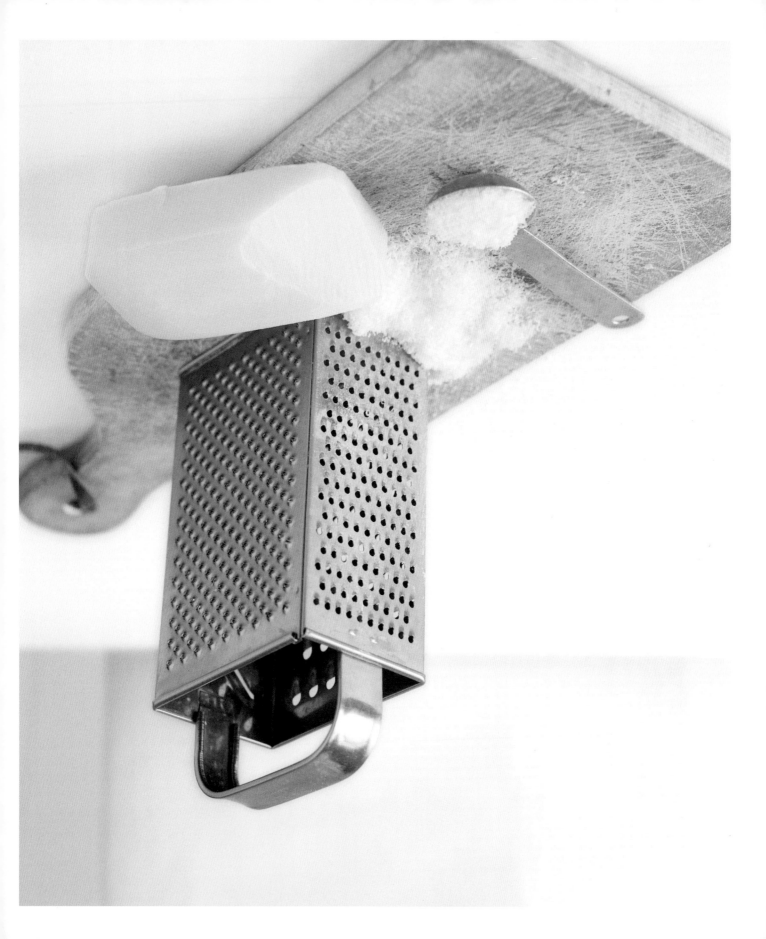

or by having a quick look in the bathroom, where you may have, for example, witch hazel or aspirin.

A visit to your local health-food store and ethnic grocery will also result in some indispensable ingredients, while plant and other materials gathered during a country walk or trip to the seashore will offer more exciting options with which to experiment (but please don't take more than you need, and never remove entire plants). And these days the internet allows us to track down the most unusual ingredients with ease. Online suppliers provide the most comprehensive selection of specialist items such as emulsifiers, butters and powders. The hardest part is not getting too enthused by the choice and ordering too much.

While the 'Sourcing Ingredients' section provides an overview of useful ingredients for natural beauty products and where you might find them, the Glossary at the end of the book lists every ingredient used in our recipes, so you can easily check the function of each one and learn its INCI – that is, its internationally recognized – name.

In the 'Mastering Techniques' section, we encourage you to learn a few valuable skills that will greatly enhance your ability to make the most of your store cupboard of ingredients. Those fresh, summery herbs from your garden can be captured and preserved as infusions to be added to your recipes at any time of the year, and an understanding of the importance of preservatives and emulsifiers is essential in making effective, functional skin- or haircare. In this section we also discuss how to use specialist natural ingredients that enable you to create a more sophisticated and varied range of recipes. Making skincare at home doesn't rule out having some really great textures that look and feel like expensive, store-bought cosmetics.

As in the case of cooking, when you're making handmade cosmetics it's vital to remember the principles of working safely, and you must follow straightforward rules of hygiene; so we have included tips to ensure that the recipes come out right each time. Most of these pointers are common sense, but it's easy to get carried away with an idea and neglect the basics. So please study the page devoted to 'Considering Storage and Safety', which will help you to make the products safely, then keep and use them effectively.

Once you have mastered the techniques and made a few trial recipes, you will no doubt want to show off what you have made. In the 'Finishing Touches' section, we offer suggestions on how to embellish your creations so they look attractive on your bathroom shelf or dressing table, and how to package and present them as gorgeous gifts. Do remember, however, that although these recipes have been thoroughly tested, they are just for personal use and should not be sold, as the regulations and legislation for selling cosmetics are very strict.

The recipes in this book are intended to provide both guidance and inspiration as you begin to craft your own natural beauty products. They are the result of our years of experience in the cosmetics industry and in teaching homemade beauty classes, and we hope that, in passing them on, we tempt you to have a go – and have fun.

A NOTE ON CONVERSIONS

When following the recipes, stick to one set of measurements, either metric or imperial. Many recipes require small quantities of ingredients, so in some cases it may be easier to measure out teaspoons rather than use digital scales. Teaspoon and tablespoon quantities given in parentheses are the US versions. Where only one measurement in teaspoons or tablespoons is given, this is the UK measurement, which is a bit bigger than its US equivalent: 5 UK teaspoons/tablespoons are equivalent to 6 US teaspoons/tablespoons, so readers in the United States will need to add a little more. However, in the case of very small quantities (say, 1–2 teaspoons), the difference between UK and US teaspoons is negligible.

BEFORE YOU BEGIN

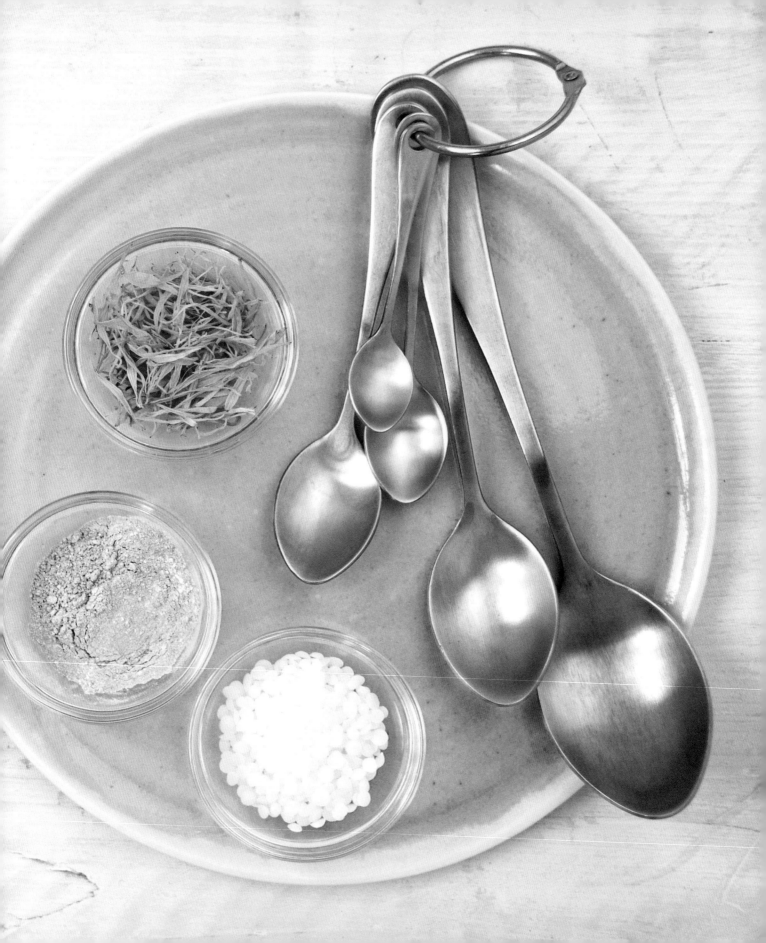

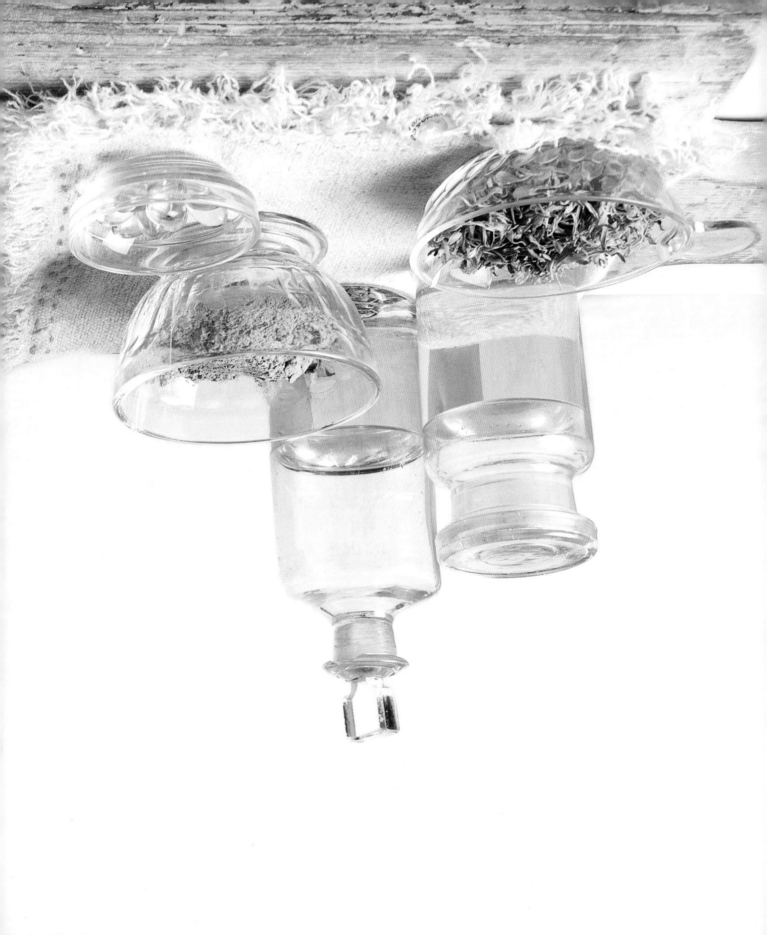

Sourcing Ingredients

IT'S REMARKABLE HOW MANY OF THE INGREDIENTS IN AN AVERAGE
KITCHEN CUPBOARD OR BATHROOM CABINET CAN BE USED TO MAKE
A VARIETY OF HANDMADE COSMETICS. A TRIP TO THE HEALTH-FOOD
STORE OR ETHNIC GROCERS WILL PROVIDE SOME EXCELLENT
ADDITIONAL MATERIALS, LEAVING JUST A FEW ITEMS THAT ARE BEST
OBTAINED FROM A SPECIALIST ONLINE SUPPLIER. AND DON'T FORGET
THE DIVERSE PLANT MATERIALS THAT CAN BE SOURCED FROM THE
GARDEN, SEASHORE, HEDGEROW OR EVEN A WINDOW BOX. THIS
SECTION SUGGESTS WHAT INGREDIENTS TO LOOK FOR AND WHERE TO
FIND THEM, AND OUTLINES THEIR USES IN NATURAL SKIN- AND HAIRCARE.

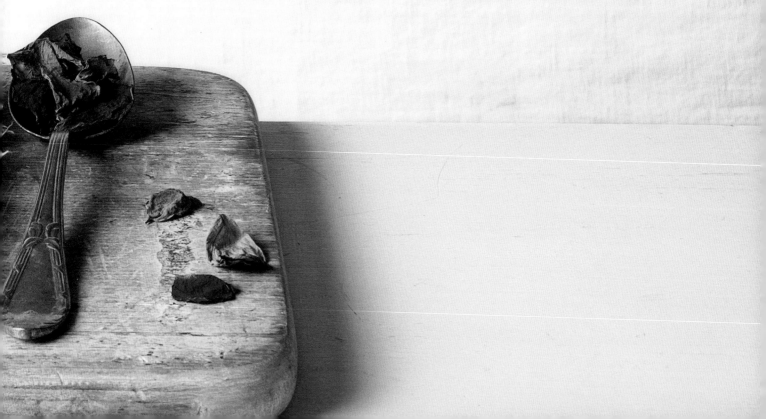

In the Health-Food Store

These days, it's possible to find a health-food store in most towns, whatever their size. These stores are convenient locations for stocking up on some staple ingredients, as well as purchasing a few more unusual items for cosmetic recipes. The staff are usually knowledgeable, and this can be very helpful when you're searching for or experimenting with new ingredients. Feel free to seek advice when trying out something a bit different, as some of the intriguing products may at first seem unlikely raw materials for the recipes you plan to make.

You'll discover a wide selection of essential oils for adding scent as well as beneficial properties to your recipes (see pages 24–25 for more information on these oils and guidelines on how to use them effectively and safely). In addition, the range of grains, seeds and powders more commonly used in food products is surprisingly just as useful in skincare. Many of the ingredients that you might add to a smoothie or your morning muesli are equally good in a cosmetic product such as a scrub or a wash-off cleansing powder. The extensive selection of vitamins and nutritional supplements is especially useful for adding powerful antioxidants and anti-ageing properties – as you might find in premium-brand skincare – to your own creations.

USEFUL INGREDIENTS

- **Aloe vera juice:** Well known for its moisturizing, anti-inflammatory and skin-soothing properties; and particularly useful as an aftersun treatment.
- **Avocado oil:** Rich in vitamin E, the oil is widely used for its regenerative and moisturizing properties to improve the condition of hair, skin and nails.
- **Beeswax:** A natural thickening agent that lends the skin a protective, moisture-retaining surface.
- **Chia seeds and omega sprinkles:** Rich in omega-3 fatty acids; they make an unusual and nourishing exfoliating ingredient in scrubs and skin polishes.
- **Coconut water:** A delicious drink and a refreshing and hydrating alternative to using water, as shown in our Skin-Brightening Tropical Toner recipe (see page 60).
- **Dead Sea salt:** A mineral-rich exfoliating ingredient, used for centuries in scrubs and bath products for its ability to help relaxation and treat minor skin conditions.
- **Epsom salts:** A traditional crystal-like powder containing magnesium, often used in bath products to help detox the body and ease stiff muscles.
- **Essential oils:** Such as geranium, lavender and tea tree; these oils are used extensively for their fragrance as well as reputed therapeutic properties.

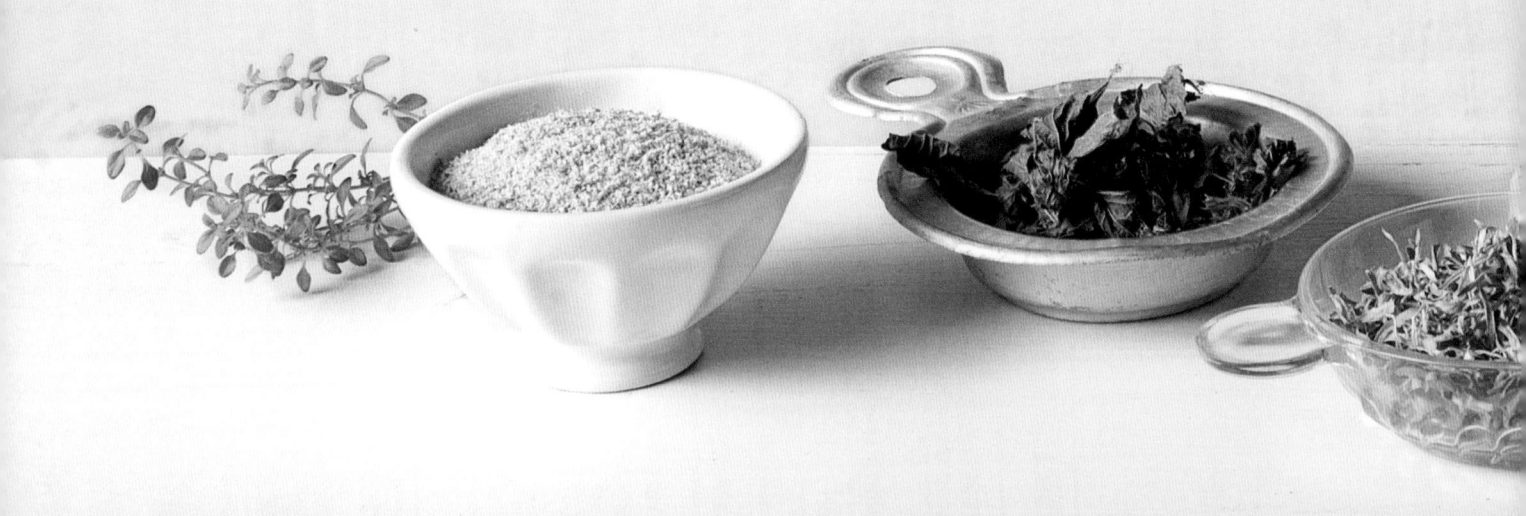

- **Grapefruit seed extract (GSE):** A natural preservative used to prolong the shelf life of many products that would otherwise have to be used immediately or kept in the fridge for only a few days.
- **Kaolin** (*white clay*)**:** A highly effective base for face masks on account of its ability to absorb impurities and toxins from the skin.
- **Liquorice root:** Used as a traditional remedy for digestive problems, but owing to its anti-inflammatory properties it's beneficial for troubled and dry skin and can help to even skin tone.
- **Manuka honey:** Produced only in New Zealand by bees pollinating the native manuka bush. It's well known for its exceptional anti-inflammatory and healing properties. We've used it in both our Gentle Dispersing Face Scrub/Mask (see page 77) and Dispersing Body Scrub (see page 107).
- **Natural soap:** Grated unperfumed soap can be used as a cleansing ingredient in bath and foot powders.
- **Oat bran and rice bran powders:** More commonly associated with breakfast cereals, these coarse-textured powders have natural cleansing properties, and are ideal for use in bath soaks and gentle facial scrubs. You can also use porridge oats by simply blitzing them in a coffee grinder to obtain the ideal texture.
- **Rice bran oil:** A light, vitamin-rich oil that is a useful addition to skincare oils, creams and lotions, protecting against dryness and skin-damaging free radicals.
- **Sodium bicarbonate** (*baking soda*)**:** A multi-purpose powder generally used for its cleaning properties. Combined with citric acid (see overleaf), it is an essential ingredient in bath bombs and effervescing powders.
- **Sweet almond oil:** A multi-purpose light, vitamin-rich and quickly absorbed skin-conditioning oil, used in creams, lotions and massage oils; often used as carrier oil to dilute essential and other potent oils prior to topical application.
- **Vitamins, minerals and supplements:** Health-food stores are the place to shop for these valuable additives. Their selection is expansive, and options range from well-known supplements such as evening primrose oil and ginseng to other more unusual ingredients, such as chlorella, gotu kola, astragalus and rhodiola (which all feature in our recipes). These natural actives, available in capsule or tablet form, can be added easily to boost the efficacy of creams and other leave-on products.

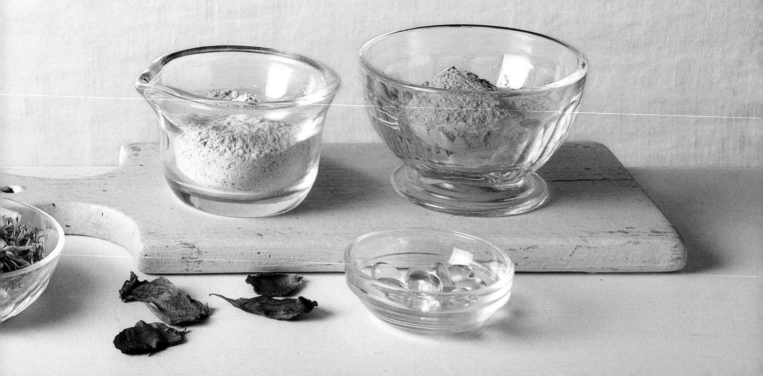

In the Ethnic Grocery

As a result of their diverse and multicultural populations, many towns and cities benefit from being home to ethnic grocery stores. You may expect to see a vast array of colourful spices on offer – often a selection far greater than available in even huge out-of-town supermarkets – but you're equally likely to be delighted by the exciting ingredients you discover on a more extensive search of these individual local shops: not just unusual fruits and vegetables, but also oils and exotic flavoured waters and teas. All present enticing possibilities for making your own cosmetic products.

You'll often find that our favourite ethnic grocery ingredients are surprisingly inexpensive, so be sure to stock up when you're there.

USEFUL INGREDIENTS

- **Argan oil:** A nut oil from Morocco. Closely related to the olive, the argan nut is more difficult to harvest, hence its elevated price in comparison to many more common cooking oils. Argan oil is used as an anti-ageing ingredient in creams, lotions and facial oils on account of its antioxidant properties and high vitamin E and fatty acid content.
- **Citric acid:** A natural cleaning agent and pH modifier (see page 41), traditionally used in brewing and wine-making. It is an essential ingredient in bath bombs and any fizzing bath powder, creating the 'fizz' when combined with sodium bicarbonate (baking soda; see page 15).
- **Coconut milk:** Used widely in Southeast Asian cuisine for curries, desserts and drinks; also makes a great cleansing and conditioning ingredient for your cosmetic recipes when mixed in the water phase.
- **Green tea:** Well known for its high vitamin content and antioxidant properties, and widely seen as a healthy option both as a hot drink and as an ingredient in soft drinks, smoothies and desserts. In skincare, green tea infusions can be used in the water phase to add enhanced anti-ageing properties to recipes. The loose tea is generally of a higher quality and preferable to tea bags.

- **Herbs and spices:** Whether your chosen ethnic store has its origin in India, the Middle East, the West Indies or China, it will be the place to stock up on all those herbs and spices that you need for both cooking and cosmetic recipes, for use in infusions in particular. You'll find the packs are larger than the supermarket versions, but offer much better value.
- **Mint water:** As in the case of the more familiar rose and orange flower waters (see below), mint water can be used as part of a water phase in a cosmetic recipe. Delightfully refreshing, it makes a lovely addition to facial toners and body lotions and washes.
- **Orange flower water:** A floral water used extensively in the Middle East, where its distinctive scent gives a wonderful flavour to fruit salads in particular. Obtained by distillation from the blossom of the bitter orange tree, it is also used in drinks, biscuits and desserts. We like to use this delicately aromatic ingredient in the water phase of many of our recipes; it is invaluable in facial toners, creams and lotions.
- **Rose water:** A by-product of the production of rose oil, and another major ingredient in Middle Eastern cuisine, where its delicate fragrance enhances sweets, desserts, cakes and fruit salads. We use rose water in the water phase of many of our recipes to give a subtle aroma and added freshness. It can also be used on its own as a quick, hydrating facial spritz.
- **Unrefined coconut oil:** A popular ingredient in a variety of healthy cuisine recipes, whether used for frying or baking, or in dressings and desserts. It is enjoying a recent revival as a beauty favourite on account of its use as an instant hair treatment, but we also like to add it to body butters and creams.
- **Yoghurt:** A staple of the ethnic grocer; where possible, we prefer to buy the Greek-style thick yoghurt. As a radiance-enhancing and line-smoothing ingredient for instant fresh face masks or even as a hydrating quick fix for sunburn, it deserves to become a permanent fixture in your fridge.

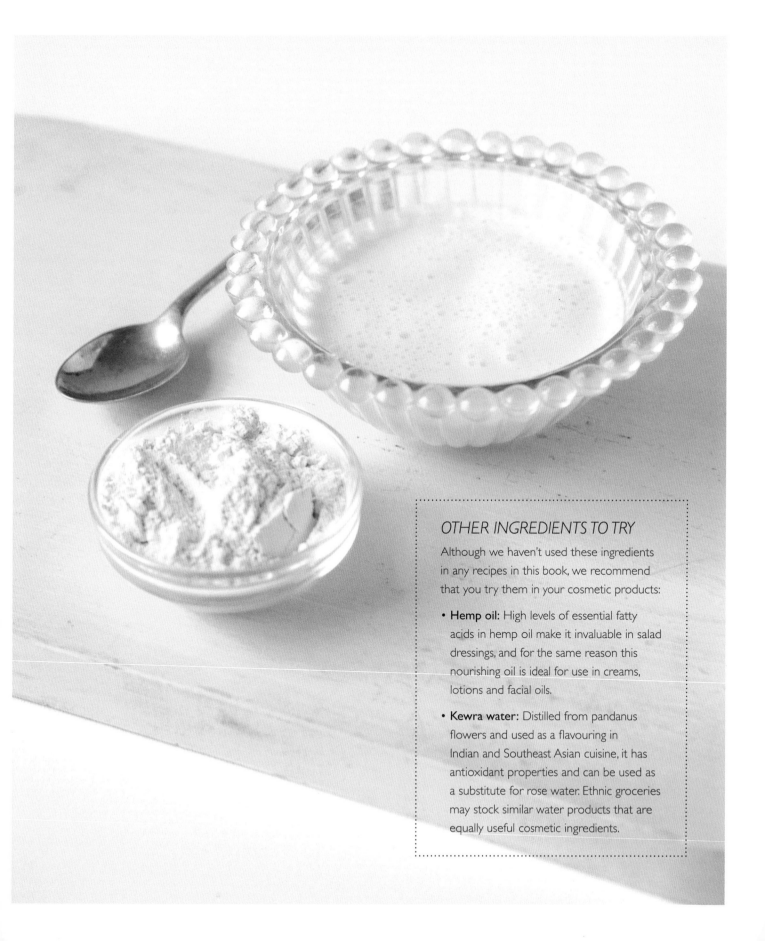

OTHER INGREDIENTS TO TRY

Although we haven't used these ingredients
in any recipes in this book, we recommend
that you try them in your cosmetic products:

• **Hemp oil:** High levels of essential fatty
acids in hemp oil make it invaluable in salad
dressings, and for the same reason this
nourishing oil is ideal for use in creams,
lotions and facial oils.

• **Kewra water:** Distilled from pandanus
flowers and used as a flavouring in
Indian and Southeast Asian cuisine, it has
antioxidant properties and can be used as
a substitute for rose water. Ethnic groceries
may stock similar water products that are
equally useful cosmetic ingredients.

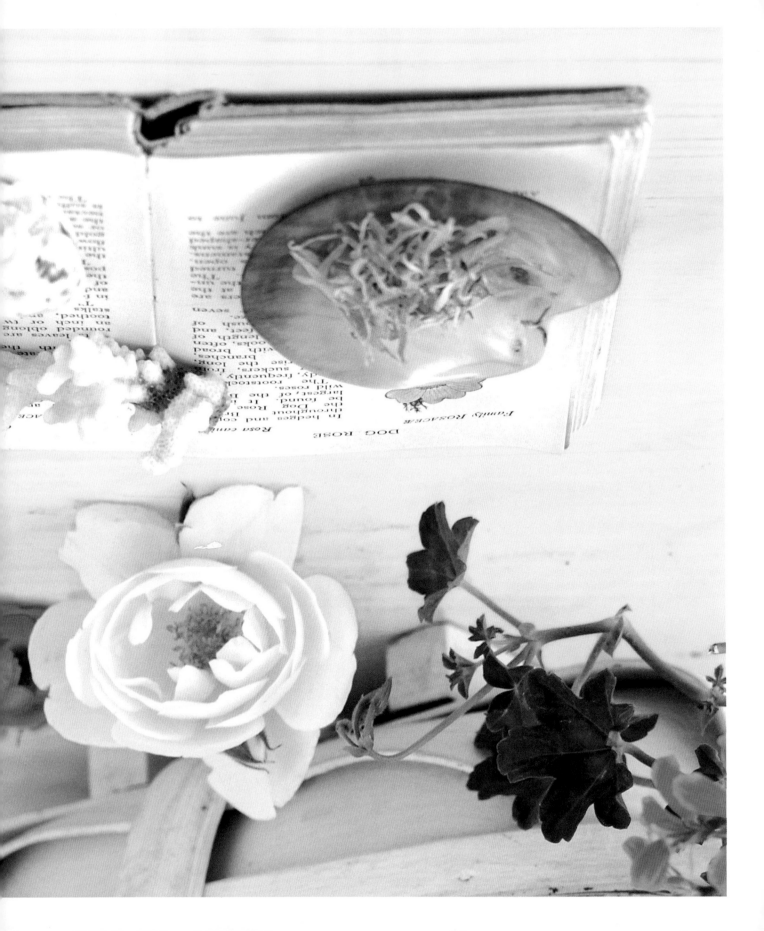

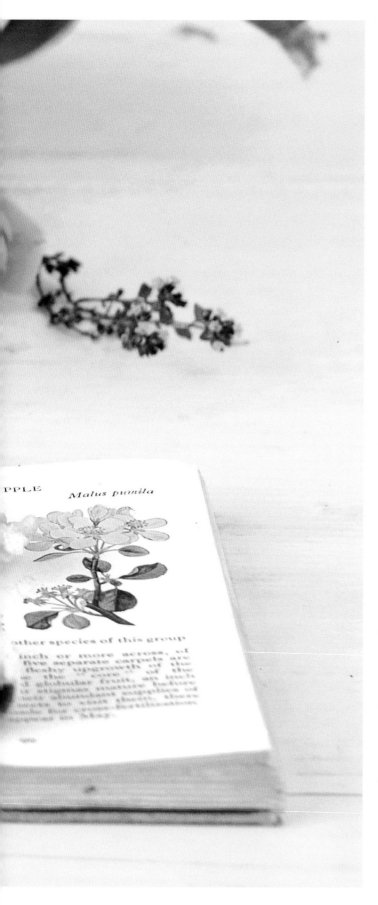

Exploring the Garden, Hedgerow and Seashore

Our gardens, the countryside and the seashore all offer treasures that can be used in cosmetic recipes. Even if your garden extends to only a small paved area, or you have just a window box, you have the opportunity to grow a small but useful selection of plants with which you can experiment. If you're an organic gardener, you also have the satisfaction of knowing that anything you grow is free of pesticides and as fresh as possible.

Our hedges contain diverse plants, trees and shrubs, which all too often we fail to notice. There is a natural larder for our skin- and haircare ingredients, but be sure not to deplete the native environment when you go foraging, whether in the country or by the sea, and never remove a plant by its roots. Please take only what you need and leave plenty for others to enjoy.

USEFUL INGREDIENTS

- **Comfrey:** A less common garden herb than those listed below, traditionally used for its healing properties owing to the presence in its leaves of allantoin, which reduces inflammation. Use a glycerine infusion (see page 37) to incorporate this benefit into creams and lotions; it's ideal for acne-prone skin.
- **Culinary herbs** (*lemon balm, marjoram, mint, rosemary, sage, thyme*): Can be used fresh or dried in bath powders and salts, but also make effective infusions that can be added to creams or lotions to deliver their special properties.
- **Dried calendula** (*marigold*) **petals:** Have a pretty orange colour and can be used in a similar way to dried rose petals (see overleaf). The petals retain their colour well after drying.
- **Dried lavender flowers:** A versatile ingredient, with a lovely scent that is deeply relaxing and can be helpful in promoting sleep. The flowers can be incorporated as a calming element in sleep pillows and soothing masks, but

also give bath powders, bath bombs and powder cleansers a natural and visual lift.

- **Dried rose petals:** A good decorative ingredient in bath bombs, adding colour and texture; can also be added to powder products such as our Japanese Gentle Exfoliating Cleansing Powder (see page 54). Red petals hold their colour better than pink, which go brown quickly.
- **Elderflowers:** The scented white flowers of the elder tree or shrub (native to most of Europe) are well known for their use in a refreshing cordial. Fresh or dried, they can also be used in face masks and creams for their skin-brightening properties. If elderflowers are not available, we have suggested alternative ingredients in recipes.
- **Nettles:** Nettles are antioxidant, contain antimicrobial activity and have long been associated with the treatment of scalp problems. Their sting disappears once they're cooked, so add a water infusion of nettles to shampoo and scalp conditioner recipes, or use it as a hair rinse.
- **Sand:** A walk on warm, fine beach sand exfoliates your bare feet, so try adding a small amount of clean, washed sand to an oil, gel or cream base for an instant foot scrub.

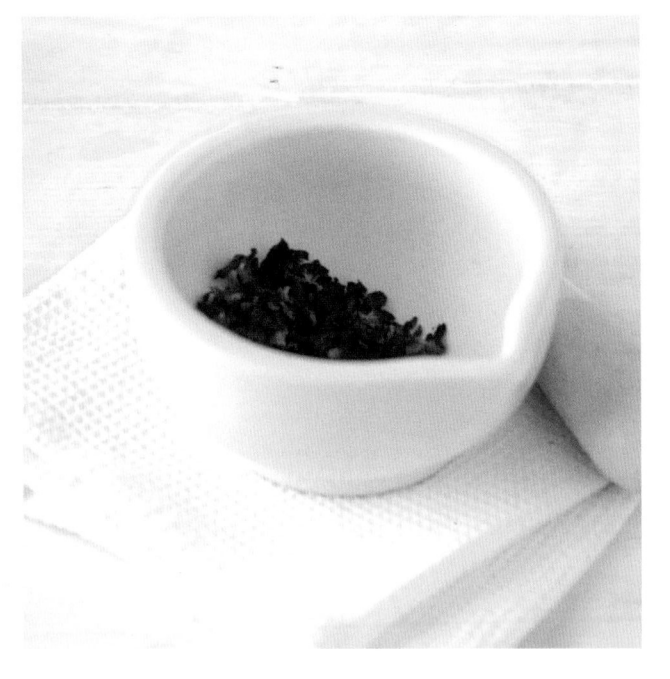

HOW TO DRY PETALS

Select fresh flowers in full bloom from your garden or window box. Pluck the petals gently from their base. Avoid picking browning petals, and make sure the petals are not damp with dew, as any moisture could cause them to rot.

Arrange a single layer of petals on top of a paper towel placed on a tray. Leave in a warm, dry spot out of direct sunlight – a shelf in an airing cupboard is ideal. Air-drying petals takes a few days. Turn the petals over at least once during that time. Wait until they are crispy-dry before using them. Store in an airtight container, away from direct light and heat.

- **Scented geranium/pelargonium:** The leaves can be used as an epicurean delight in sorbets, or infused in sugar for baking and in drinks. Add dried leaves to herb pillows and bath powders, salts and scrubs for texture and a hint of aroma. The essential oil of this plant is used extensively in aromatherapy and skincare for its various benefits.
- **Sea lavender:** A sand-loving plant with long-lasting, bright lilac flowers. It's used as an anti-ageing ingredient in cosmetics, and is also known for its anti-inflammatory and firming action. A glycerine infusion of the leaves can be made to utilize the beneficial properties of the plant.
- **Sea shells:** We don't suggest that you use shells as a recipe ingredient, but the range of sizes and shapes makes them fun to use imaginatively to decorate your cosmetic gifts.
- **Seaweed:** Its texture and mineral-rich content make dried seaweed an excellent ingredient in body scrubs. You could also add fresh or dried seaweed directly to your bath, along with Dead Sea salt (see page 14), as a detoxifying treatment. Always wash seaweed thoroughly before use.
- **Yarrow:** A common, unassuming white-flowered plant, the wild version of garden achillea. An infusion made from the whole plant is helpful in treating dry skin.

In the Kitchen and Bathroom

The kitchen cupboard and bathroom cabinet will yield a surprisingly large number of useful ingredients for home-made skin- and haircare. (And you probably have most of the tools you'll need in your kitchen, too; see page 28). So start by searching your cupboards for items that you already own and can put to good use (provided that they are not past their use-by date, of course). By adding just a few specialist ingredients to the versatile items below, you can start practising and gain experience in making a wide selection of recipes.

USEFUL INGREDIENTS

- **Acai berry juice:** A delicious drink packed with high levels of antioxidants, vitamins and minerals; its addition to skincare products such as spray toners is a great way of incorporating these valuable ingredients.
- **Beer:** Has a long history of use in hair products, and at one time was often touted as an active constituent of shampoos. It adds shine, volume and condition, and in the past was used as an inexpensive styling lotion, applied prior to setting the hair with rollers, clips or curlers. Try to use beer that has been made by traditional methods, rather than a mass-produced alternative.
- **Dried milk powder:** With supermarkets open 24/7 these days, we are perhaps less likely than previous generations to have dried milk powder in the cupboard. However, as well as being a standby for a cup of tea or coffee, it makes an effective skin conditioner in bath powders owing to its vitamin, mineral and protein content.
- **Gelatine:** A setting agent, traditionally used to thicken desserts and fillings. It's a by-product of the meat industry, but there is a vegetarian option, so be sure to check the manufacturer's ingredient listing carefully if you prefer to use non-animal products. Available in sheet form, as we've used to help set a face mask (see page 83), or as a powder version. Usage instructions will vary, so always read the information on the pack.
- **Glycerine:** A clear, slightly syrupy humectant (a substance used to keep things moist), frequently used as a cosmetic ingredient because of its ability to hold moisture to the skin; also used in foods and pharmaceuticals. Beneficial herbs, roots, flowers and even seaweed can be steeped in a preserved glycerine-and-water mix (see page 37) to provide a range of naturally active ingredients for adding to creams and lotions.
- **Olive oil:** A kitchen staple, this inexpensive and versatile ingredient can be used as a base oil for massage, or as an emollient in creams and lotions. We've used it in a face mask for dry or mature skin (see page 78).
- **Oranges and lemons:** Citrus fruits have long been associated with cleaning, and lemon in particular has a naturally brightening and bleaching effect. The scent of lemon is synonymous with cleanliness and freshness. Fresh lemon juice can be used in a hair rinse, and we've found the zest of lemons and oranges to be beneficial in an exfoliating hand scrub (see page 114).
- **Sea salt:** Contains a high level of naturally occurring minerals (refined salt loses many of these trace elements in processing), and is both detoxifying and exfoliating to the skin; also helps to heal minor skin conditions. It can be added to baths or used in body and hand scrubs.
- **Soluble aspirin:** Not only a good headache treatment, but also an excellent ingredient for face masks and clarifiers because it can help to soothe and brighten the skin.
- **Vinegar:** A natural cleaner as well as a kitchen staple, traditionally diluted in water to clean and descale windows and surfaces. We've added cider vinegar to our hair rinse recipe (see page 129) in tribute to its long association with adding shine to the hair.
- **Witch hazel:** Traditionally used for treating insect bites, stings and minor irritations, it has many uses in cosmetics on account of its astringent properties, hence its inclusion in facial toners and cooling foot sprays. It also helps to bind together the other ingredients in bath bombs.
- **Xanthan gum:** A natural food thickening additive derived from corn sugar; can also be used to thicken and stabilize cosmetic creams and lotions. Pre-mixing it with glycerine makes it easier to disperse into water.

On the Internet

In recent years the internet has revolutionized how we shop, and has allowed niche companies to thrive by serving very specific customer needs. The recipes in this book cannot all be made without purchases from online specialist suppliers to supplement store-bought ingredients.

Primarily, the internet will provide the most specialized items on your shopping list, including preservatives, butters, emulsifiers and specialist oils. Online suppliers will also have a wider selection of essential oils than your local health-food store, but always check the pricing, as regular deals on the high street can work out cheaper for more common items. The internet is also the best place to search for product containers (see page 30).

USEFUL INGREDIENTS

Note that we explain how to use many of these ingredients in the 'Mastering Techniques' section; see pages 38–43.

Emulsifiers

• **Emulsifying Wax BP:** A blended emulsifying wax that's very easy to use and effective in emulsifying water and oil phases in creams; it also has a thickening effect that is useful in creating butters.
• **ESP Organic SafeEmuls SCA:** A naturally derived material from coconut oil, sugar and aloe extract, used to emulsify creams and lotions. It creates a mousse-like texture, and can be used on its own or in combination with beeswax.
• **Olivem 1000:** A natural emulsifier derived from olive oil, featured in several recipes in this book on account of its ease of use and excellent spreadability and moisturization properties.

Butters and Clays

• **Cocoa butter:** Melts at close to body temperature, making it an ideal choice for inclusion in salves and body butters, as well as bath melts. It is not advised for use in facial products because it can encourage acne.
• **Shea butter:** Also known as karité butter; a particularly effective moisturizer because it contains so many fatty acids, which are needed to retain skin moisture and elasticity. This attribute also makes it an excellent additive for face and body creams and lotions, and body butters.
• **Coloured clays:** As well as the more common kaolin, a white clay (see page 15), you can choose pink or green clays, which work in the same way but also add colour and variety to your recipes. We use clay in face masks to thicken the product and draw impurities out of the skin.

Examples of Specialist Oils

• **Borage oil:** Also known as starflower oil; high in omega-3 and omega-6 fatty acids, it is used in anti-ageing skincare, where it helps to tone and restore suppleness.
• **Rosehip oil:** Obtained from rosehip seeds, this oil is recommended for acne scarring. Excellent in facial oils and creams, it's also used as an anti-ageing treatment to help reduce wrinkles and fine lines.

Specialist Ingredients

• **Lamesoft PO 65:** Naturally derived from coconut and sunflower oils; it's used in combination with Plantapon LGC (see below) to thicken foaming wash-off products, as well as adding moisturizing properties.
• **Plantapon LGC:** A natural surfactant derived from coconut oil and sugar, it has excellent foaming properties while being mild in use. When incorporated in natural shampoos, it contributes to hair softness and improves dry-combing properties; also recommended for face and body washes and bath soaks.
• **Polysorbate 20:** Used to combine essential oils in bath oils, cream preparations and shower gels or shampoos; also mild to the skin.
• **Sucragel CF:** A multi-purpose, naturally derived material used to obtain crystal-clear, waterless gels (see page 43); can also be used to make lotions and creams by adding an oil phase followed by a water phase.
• **Tin oxide:** A compound more commonly used in colour cosmetics or ceramics. We've used it in our Nail Buffer recipe (see page 116) for its ultra-fine abrasive qualities.

BUYER BEWARE!

As in the case of all online shopping, it's easy to get carried away, so check what you really need before ordering, and don't allow yourself to be seduced into buying unnecessary items. Buy from reputable sites only.

You'll find that raw materials are cheaper to buy in bulk, but bear in mind that they also have a shelf life, and most internet suppliers have an additional charge for carriage that is generally based on weight. So it's sensible to purchase only what you calculate you'll need for the recipes you're planning now.

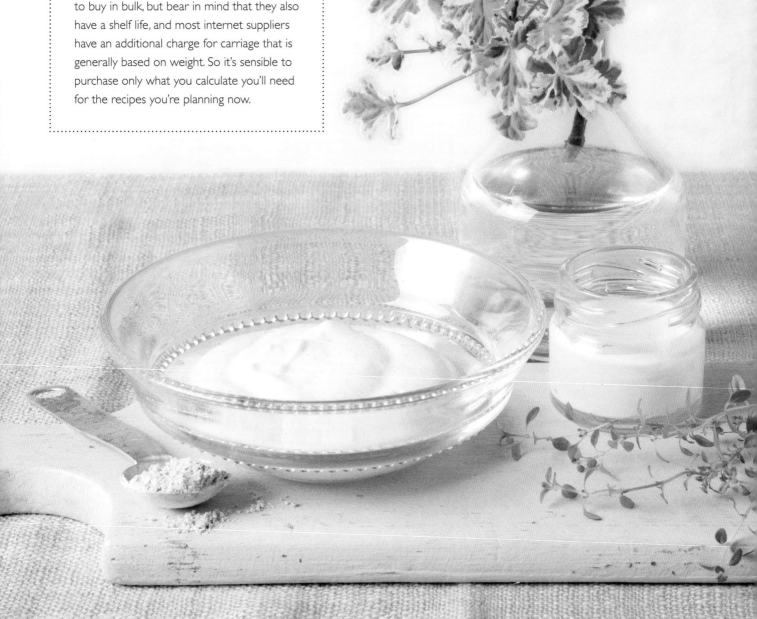

Essential Oils

Essential oils are a key ingredient when you're making your own skin- and haircare products, and are possibly the most exciting element. You usually add these oils as the last stage of a recipe, and they can change the fragrance and mood of a product quite dramatically.

WHAT ARE ESSENTIAL OILS?

Essential oils are not at all like the botanical, nut and seed oils that we use to build a recipe; they are volatile aromatic compounds extracted from flowers, fruits, leaves, roots and woods. Each in its own right contains numerous individual compounds that make up the characteristic essential oil we recognize from its aroma.

Different plants have greater or lesser amounts of these volatile oils in their cells, and the quality of the oil may be affected by climatic conditions and the harvest in any given year. Generally speaking, a plant with a very high oil content – such as mint, orange or eucalyptus – results in a cheaper end product. Lavender also gives a high level of oil. However, some herbs and delicate flowers such as camomile have a poor oil yield, and therefore the essential oils are extremely expensive, and are used in only tiny amounts in a perfume or cosmetic product.

EXTRACTION

Essential oils are obtained by several methods. The most common is **steam distillation**, whereby steam is passed through the plant material, such as rose petals. As the steam condenses, the aromatic essential oil in the plant material rises to the surface of the water and can then be separated off. The remaining water is the 'flower water', which has taken on a delicate aroma of the flower oil. We have used flower waters such as rose and orange flower extensively in our recipes; see, for example, the Wipe-Off Cleanser with Sucragel, Rose and Lavender on page 50.

The most expensive flower oils, such as rose absolute (as opposed to rose otto, obtained by steam distillation) and jasmine absolute, are obtained via **solvent extraction** so as not to damage the delicate petals. In this method, a solvent such as methanol is used to extract the odorous material from the plant. The yield is very low for these precious oils: for example, 100kg (220lb) of rose petals can produce as little as 500ml (17fl oz) of finished essential oil. This accounts for the very high cost and the fact that some of the most expensive oils are sold in dilution. It is important to check what dosage of oil you are buying. Rose, jasmine and camomile essential oils are typically sold as blended versions, generally at 5–10% strength in a carrier oil such as sweet almond.

USING ESSENTIAL OILS

Essential oils are very potent ingredients and should be used with care. In their undiluted state they should never be applied directly to the skin, as they can cause an allergic reaction. They should not be used in any eye products. Additionally, there are essential oils that are contraindicated for use in pregnancy. Seek advice if you are in any doubt.

Blending Oils

In each recipe, we have indicated the dosage (see the box opposite for general guidelines) and chosen the essential oils based on their therapeutic effects, having given consideration to how the oils work together. The addition of essential oils to a recipe for their beneficial effect alone may not result in a pleasant aroma, so it is worth considering how they might work together to make a harmonious scent. Learning to blend essential oils is a fascinating study, and a few simple rules will help you to get a good balance of the crucial top, middle and base notes that a perfumer considers when creating a fragrance.

The top notes lend the freshness that we often notice as the opener to a perfume, such as citrus oils of lemon and grapefruit, or herby notes from mint. These notes are the most volatile and, while good for initial impact, they fade quickly – so it's important to add middle and base notes to balance the fragrance. The flower notes tend to fall into the middle category, while woody and amber tones become the base notes that give the fragrance depth and longevity.

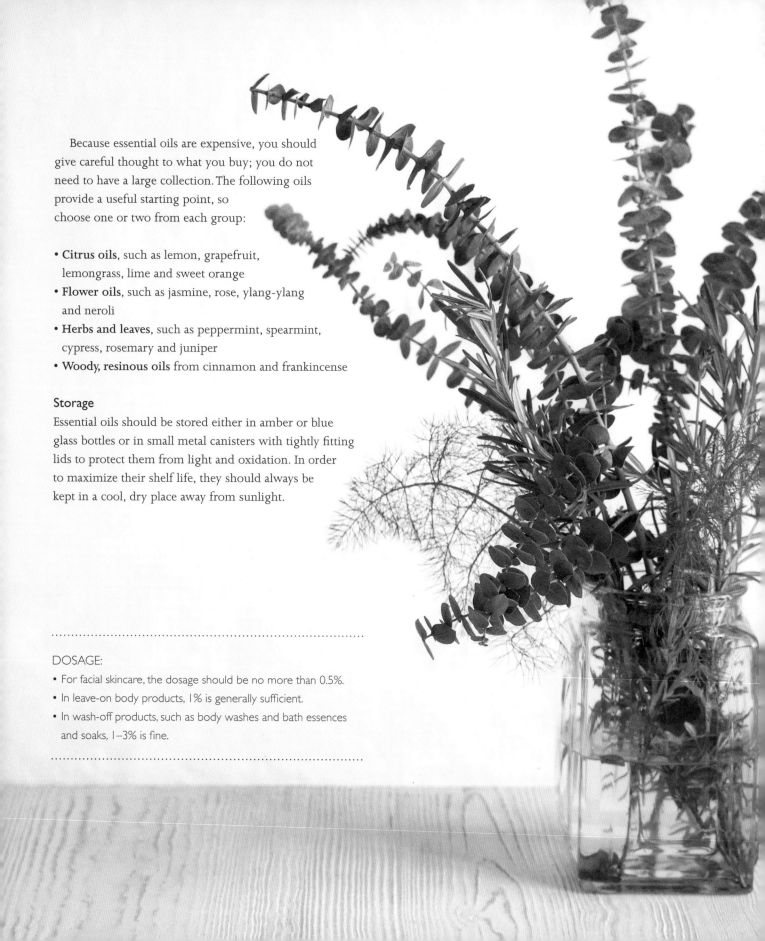

Because essential oils are expensive, you should give careful thought to what you buy; you do not need to have a large collection. The following oils provide a useful starting point, so choose one or two from each group:

- **Citrus oils**, such as lemon, grapefruit, lemongrass, lime and sweet orange
- **Flower oils**, such as jasmine, rose, ylang-ylang and neroli
- **Herbs and leaves**, such as peppermint, spearmint, cypress, rosemary and juniper
- **Woody, resinous oils** from cinnamon and frankincense

Storage

Essential oils should be stored either in amber or blue glass bottles or in small metal canisters with tightly fitting lids to protect them from light and oxidation. In order to maximize their shelf life, they should always be kept in a cool, dry place away from sunlight.

DOSAGE:
- For facial skincare, the dosage should be no more than 0.5%.
- In leave-on body products, 1% is generally sufficient.
- In wash-off products, such as body washes and bath essences and soaks, 1–3% is fine.

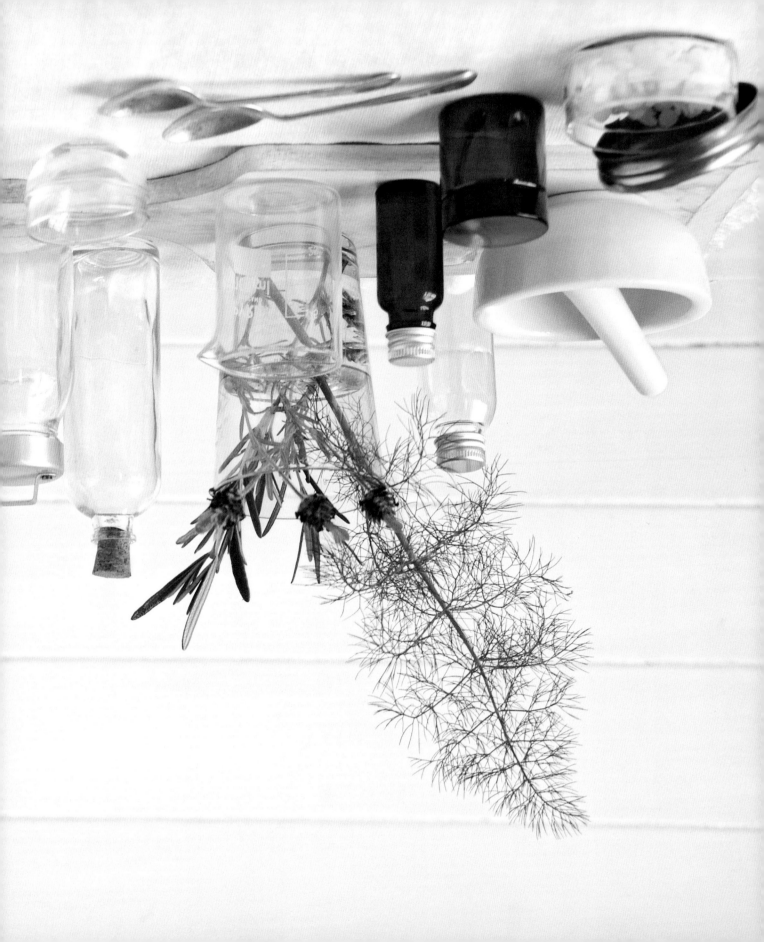

Getting Equipped

THIS MAY BE THE FIRST TIME YOU'VE TRIED MAKING YOUR OWN
SKIN- OR HAIRCARE PRODUCTS, BUT THE GOOD NEWS IS THAT
THE MAJORITY OF RECIPES IN THIS BOOK REQUIRE NO MORE THAN
THE STANDARD EQUIPMENT FOUND IN MOST KITCHENS – SO
YOU ARE UNLIKELY TO NEED TO BUY ITEMS TO GET YOU STARTED.
OUR BASIC LIST OF EQUIPMENT WILL ENABLE YOU TO MAKE THE
MOST STRAIGHTFORWARD PROJECTS; WE ALSO SUGGEST A FEW
OTHER ITEMS THAT WOULD BE WORTHWHILE INVESTMENTS.
AND WE CONSIDER THE CONTAINERS AND STORAGE OPTIONS
YOU'LL FIND USEFUL.

Basic Equipment

Because the simplest cosmetic recipes resemble easy cookery, you won't be surprised to discover that most kitchens probably contain the equipment required to make many of the products in this book:

- assortment of glasses, cups, jugs and beakers
- assortment of bottles with caps (the recipes mention if you need a pump dispenser, a spray bottle or a dropper instead)
- assortment of jars with lids (there's more on containers on page 30)
- digital scales
- heatproof glass measuring jug
- measuring spoons
- small glass bowls
- small measuring glass
- stainless steel tablespoons and teaspoons
- stainless steel saucepan

Accurate measuring of the ingredients is essential, and this requires digital scales. However, you will find that small measuring spoons can often be much easier to use. It is helpful to have a few stainless steel teaspoons when stirring and spooning ingredients. Metal utensils are more hygienic and easier to clean than plastic or wooden ones.

A small measuring glass is useful when mixing powders into liquids, such as xanthan gum in glycerine. The 'wrong' end of a teaspoon is the best way to mix such tiny amounts; or you can use a glass rod, if you have one.

It can also be invaluable to have more than one heatproof jug or beaker for the recipes that require adding multiple ingredients at different stages, and a selection of small glass bowls, dishes and jugs for measuring the ingredients in advance. This means you won't have to keep washing up as you go, so you can concentrate on checking the progress of each recipe as you make it.

Where recipes require heating a mixture over a hob (stovetop), create a simple double boiler by placing the ingredients in a heatproof jug inside a pan of simmering water. Timing is important in the recipes that require heating, so a kitchen timer (or a stopwatch on a phone) will help you to ensure that cooking times are followed.

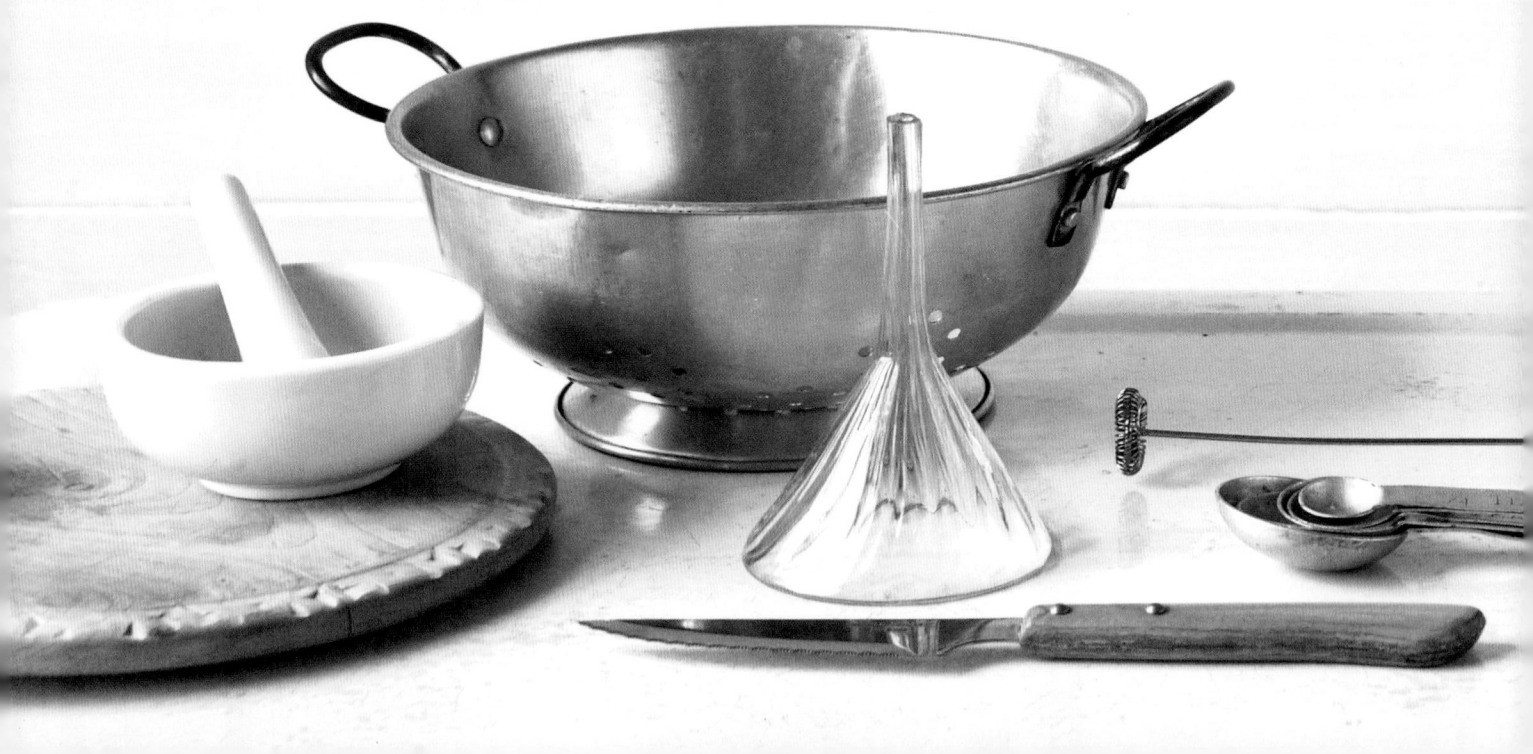

If you become well and truly hooked and find yourself making a lot of products, particularly in larger batches, it's a good idea to buy a separate set of equipment that you use exclusively for your beauty recipes.

SPECIAL EQUIPMENT

If equipment other than those items listed above is needed to make a recipe, we mention it under the heading 'Special Equipment' (after the list of ingredients for each recipe). Keen cooks, however, may already have many of these items in their kitchen.

A **stick blender** and a **thermometer** are required for numerous recipes, and should be relatively inexpensive investments if you don't have them at home. A stick blender is necessary for most of the creams and lotions, as well as some of the scrubs (if you don't have one, you can use a milk frother – of the lightweight, battery-operated kind – instead). A conventional kitchen blender is too large for many of the standard recipes, but can be used for some fresh options, where ingredients such as fruit are combined in a face mask.

Among the other items of 'special equipment' that we mention in our recipes are the following:

- **Baking tray** (*cookie sheet*): Some materials need to be pre-heated in an oven in order to sterilize them prior to use.
- **Coffee grinder:** Useful for chopping fresh herbs and dried materials into the small particles needed for most recipes.
- **Funnel:** For dispensing liquids easily. A funnel with filter paper is required to remove unwanted particles from some liquids.
- **Large mixing bowl:** To use as a water bath to cool liquids down quickly prior to adding final, delicate ingredients such as preservative (see page 66). The bowl is half-filled with ice-cold water to reduce speedily the temperature of the ingredients in a heatproof jug or bowl placed inside.
- **Pestle and mortar:** For grinding tablets into powder. Generally, a small version is the easiest to use.
- **Plastic pipette:** Where stronger liquid ingredients such as essential oils do not have a dropper top, a plastic pipette can be used as a dispenser. A pipette is also required for making a Sucragel base (see page 43).

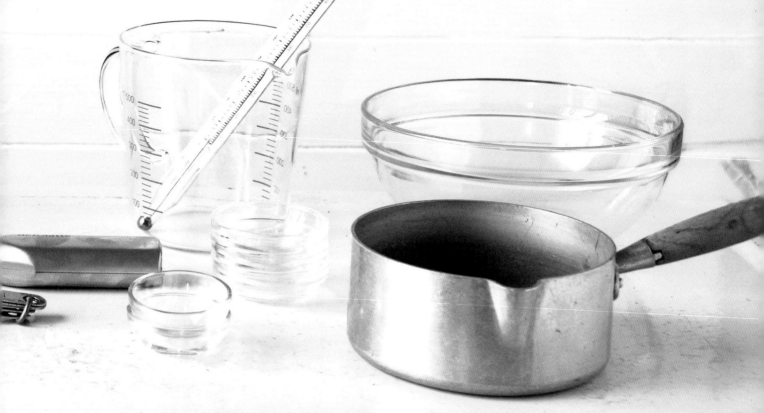

Containers and Storage

Once you've mastered some techniques (see the next section) and made a few recipes, you'll need to think about how to store your cosmetic products to ensure that you get the best from them. You'll also want to show off your work; the right container will enhance the look of the recipes you have made (see 'Adding the Finishing Touch', page 138).

SELECTING THE RIGHT CONTAINER

First, it's important to pick an appropriate container for your recipe. We discuss safety issues on page 44, but there are other points to consider.

Size Matters

Bear in mind the size of the batch you are making: a small product, such as an eye cream or a lip balm, will need a suitably small container. Similarly, a body cream or a bath product will require a larger container than a facial product. In general, it's best to make an amount of product that matches its ideal duration of use (which we indicate under the heading 'Safe Storage' in the ingredients box for each recipe), so that you don't have far more than you can use over a period of weeks or months. In this way, the product will be fresh and used at its optimum. Choosing the right size of packaging will also prevent a possible large airspace in the container if it is underfilled, which could allow some degree of unwelcome oxidation and result in the loss of quality of the product.

If the Cap Fits …

The chosen container needs to be secure and leak-proof, and should have a tight-fitting lid to ensure the maximum shelf life for your recipe. Always check that the closure matches the container (see more on this below), and remember that cosmetic jars often come with a shive. This usually takes the form of a flat plastic disc that sits under the lid in order to protect creams, scrubs and gels in transit and in use. Some bottles are fitted with a wad inside the cap, which is to prevent the contents from leaking if the product is left on its side or is sent through the post.

Pump It Up

Owing to their thicker consistency, creams are best suited to storage in jars; lotions work better in pump bottles. If you're using a pump closure, choose a lotion pump for thinner creams or gels that flow easily; an atomizer pump is suitable for a spray toner, foot spray or perfume. The output of a lotion pump determines how much liquid is dispensed when the pump is activated: you'll need a low output for an eye cream, a greater one for a body lotion.

NEW OR REUSE?

There are many companies online that supply a wide range of cosmetic containers and closures; see the Directory (pages 156–57) for some suggestions. Check that the closure will fit the jar or bottle you want. The neck size of a bottle should be stated. This is shown as two numbers separated by an oblique (/): for example, 24/400, where 24 is the outside diameter of the neck expressed in millimetres; 400 refers to the thread style of the bottle neck. The closure you select should have the same bottle-neck reference, so as long as you match the sizes, the two elements will fit and your product will not leak.

Glass, Plastic or Metal

If you have some pretty jars and bottles that you'd like to reuse, it's important to clean them thoroughly and sterilize them with hot, boiled water prior to filling. Jam jars and cosmetic jars are obvious possibilities; glass bottles should be also fine to repurpose in this way. Plastic, however, can often take on the odour or colour of what was previously stored inside, and therefore may not be suitable. As a general rule, plastic containers should be used only if new. For obvious safety reasons, products for use in the shower should be stored in plastic bottles and, for ease of use, should ideally have flip-tops or pump dispensers.

You may find some aluminium (aluminum) tins that make good containers for wax-based balms or powders. But, in general, metal is not suitable for use with most liquids or products that contain water.

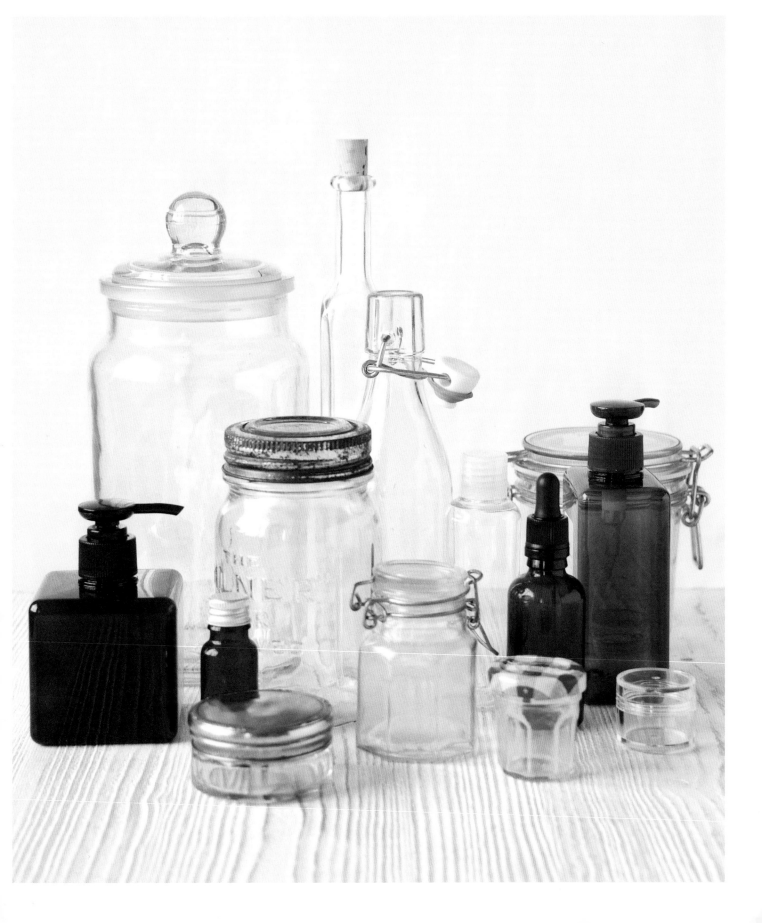

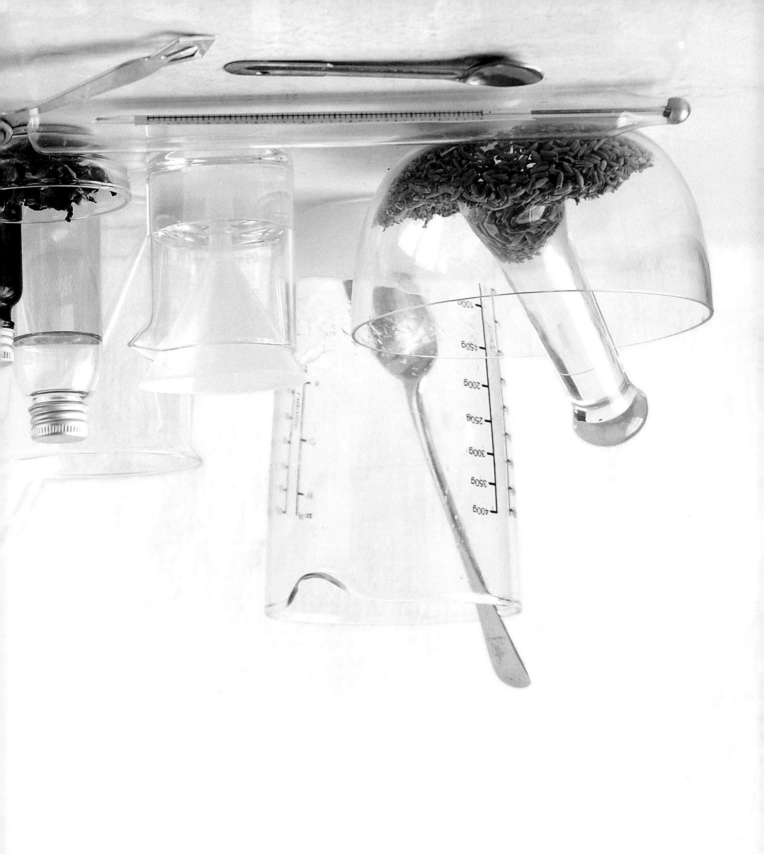

Mastering Techniques

MAKING YOUR OWN BEAUTY PRODUCTS REQUIRES SKILLS THAT WOULD BE FAMILIAR TO ANYONE WHO ENJOYS BEING CREATIVE IN THE KITCHEN. HOWEVER, THERE ARE A FEW SPECIALIZED TECHNIQUES, OUTLINED IN THE FOLLOWING PAGES, THAT SHOULD PROVIDE YOU WITH THE BUILDING BLOCKS TO MAKE A PROFESSIONAL AND SAFE COLLECTION OF COSMETIC PRODUCTS FOR FACE, BODY AND HAIR. IN THIS SECTION WE ALSO DESCRIBE HOW TO USE SPECIALIST NATURAL INGREDIENTS, AND SUMMARIZE THE POINTS YOU NEED TO THINK ABOUT WITH RESPECT TO STORAGE AND SAFETY.

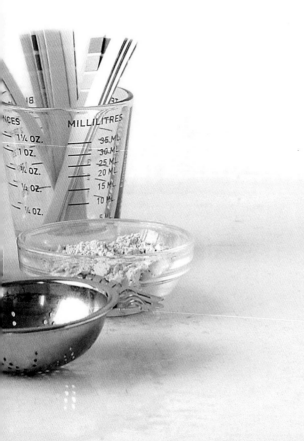

Infusions

Infusions are a way of capturing natural extracts for use in cosmetic recipes. They are very simple to make; in fact, some are virtually instant, comparable to making a cup of tea. Others involve capturing the plant material in an oil or glycerine base, which draws out the active ingredients over time – generally a few weeks.

If you have a garden or have access to wild hedgerow plants, you will find great inspiration for home-made infusions. Even a window box of herbs or a pot from the supermarket or garden centre will provide useful plant material for cosmetic infusions.

WATER-BASED INFUSIONS

Water-based infusions are a super-quick way of adding herbal, vegetable or fruit extracts to products such as water-based eye make-up removers, toners, facial sprays and face masks. See, for example, the Face Mask with Clay and Camomile Tea on page 78. The natural material can be freshly picked herbs, chopped vegetables such as cucumber, or dried green tea from the ethnic grocery. This method is particularly suited to fresh or dried leaves.

Instructions

Wash the plant material, place it in a heatproof jug or a mug, and pour over boiling water. Cover to retain the heat and vapour, and allow to infuse for around 10 minutes. Then strain the hot liquid through a tea strainer, a fine sieve (sifter) or a piece of muslin (cheesecloth) to remove all the plant material. Retain the infused liquid. If the end recipe is a face mask or any product that you intend to use immediately, there's no need to add a preservative. If you plan to keep the product for longer, we advise using a preservative such as grapefruit seed extract (see page 38).

OIL-BASED INFUSIONS

Although still quick and easy to make, infused oils are not instant like the water-based alternatives. The plant material is placed in the oil medium and left to infuse over time. Herbs, especially woody herbs such as rosemary and thyme; flowers, notably calendula (marigold) and St John's wort; roots and seaweed are ideal for oil infusions. Inexpensive carrier oils, such as olive, sunflower and sweet almond, are all suitable. In our Anti-Ageing Facial Oil on page 69, we infuse the supplements in rice bran oil.

Instructions

Clean and roughly chop the material and place it in a glass jar filled with oil, ensuring that the plant is entirely covered to avoid mould growing on the surface. Leave in a sunny window where the sealed container is exposed to light and gentle heat for around three to four weeks. Label the jar with the date so that you know when the infusion will be ready to use. The jar should be turned daily to allow the material to mix with the carrier oil.

During the infusion period you'll notice the plant changing the colour of the carrier oil; this is an indication that the process is working. When ready, strain the contents of the jar through a fine sieve (sifter) or muslin (cheesecloth), and bottle the oil in a clean jar. Discard the plant material. Label with the completed date and the name of the plant and infusion method. As these infusions contain no water, there is no need for a preservative.

Infused oils make useful additions to creams and lotions, as well as massage oils, and cuticle and nail oils and scrubs. They should keep for up to 12 months in suitable storage conditions.

GLYCERINE INFUSIONS

Glycerine infusions allow the use of concentrated extracts in small amounts and are ideal for use in creams, lotions or any recipe where glycerine is recommended. This method – described on page 37 – is excellent for tough materials, such as roots and stems (for example, liquorice root and bladderwrack can be used in infusions if chopped finely before inclusion); many wild plants are also suitable, as well as herbs and flowers. Always check that the material you use is safe, and if you're in any doubt, use something you're sure about.

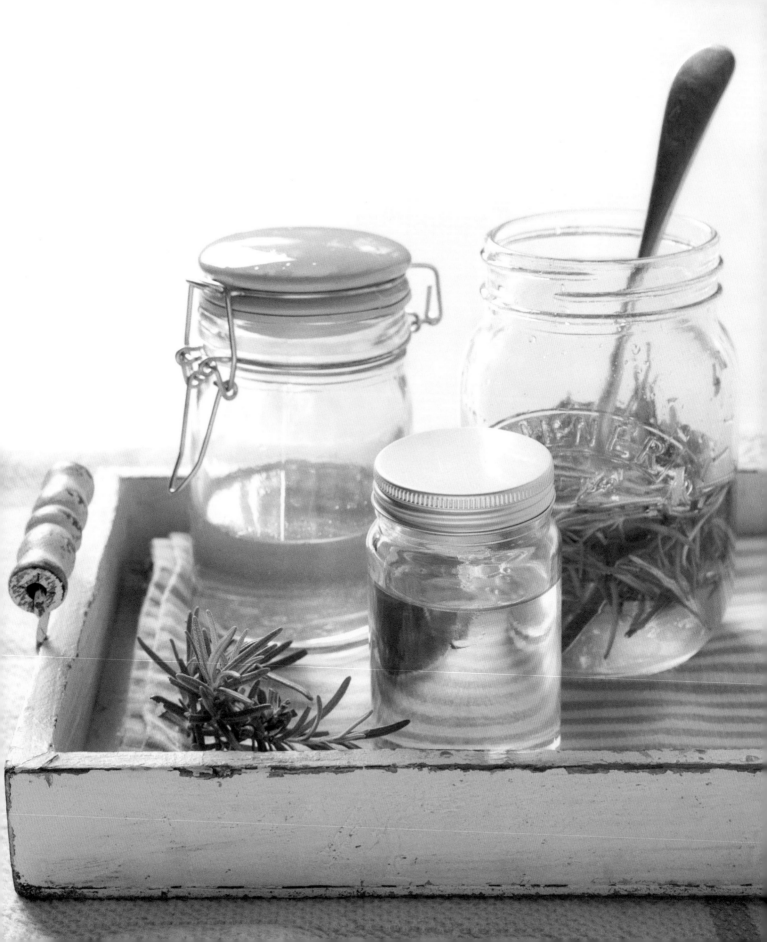

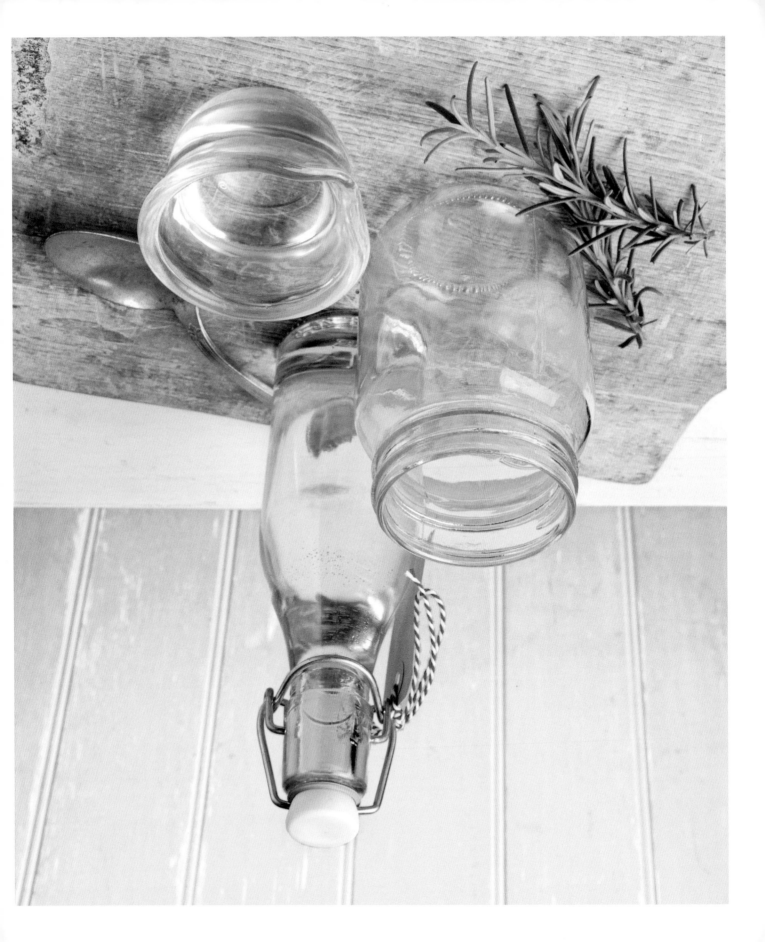

Preparing a Glycerine Infusion

First, prepare the glycerine mix by adding 70% glycerine to 30% water. For every 100ml (3½fl oz) of liquid, add 20 drops of grapefruit seed extract to preserve the liquid. Mix thoroughly. All plant material should be washed, dried and then chopped finely or ground in a coffee grinder, placed in a glass jar and covered with the glycerine mixture. As in the case of oil infusions, the plant material must be completely covered by the liquid before the sealed jar is left on a warm, sunny window ledge for around three to four weeks. Label the jar with the date, and turn it daily to ensure the material is thoroughly infused in the liquid. Check for changes in the colour of the mixture to indicate that the plant has infused in the glycerine.

Here we prepare an infusion with rosemary. This herb has antioxidant, antimicrobial and blood-stimulating properties, so the infusion can be used in foot creams, healing skin creams and haircare. See, for example, the Beer Shandy Shampoo with Lime Oil on page 126.

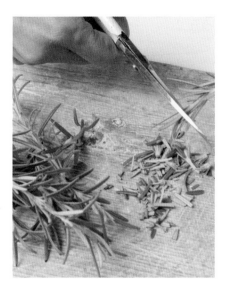

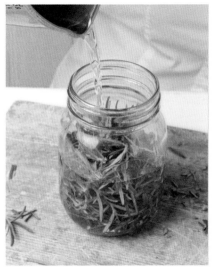

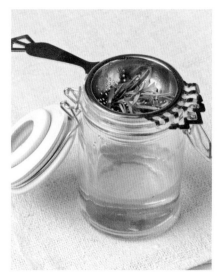

Step 1
Choose the plant material. It should be as fresh as possible and free from brown spots or any obvious discoloration. Wash and pat dry with a paper towel to remove moisture. Make up the glycerine infusion, adding 30ml (2 tbsp) of water to 70ml (4¾ tbsp) of glycerine. Add the preservative, using a ratio of 20 drops to each 100ml (3½fl oz) of the glycerine and water mixture. Mix thoroughly. Use scissors to chop the plant material into small pieces.

Step 2
Place the plant material in a glass jar, pushing down carefully in order to fit in a plentiful amount, and cover with the glycerine mixture. Ensure the plant material is fully covered by the liquid. Label the sealed jar with the date the infusion was prepared; you could also add the contents and an expected completion date four weeks from the start date. Place on a window ledge in a warm, sunny position to allow the liquid to infuse. Turn the jar daily to aid the infusion process.

Step 3
When ready to use, pour the liquid through a fine sieve (sifter) or muslin (cheesecloth) into a clean jar, cover with a tight-fitting lid, and label again with the date and contents. Glycerine infusions should keep for up to 12 months in suitable storage conditions.

Remember! *Although the glycerine infusion is preserved, you will still need to add preservative to any recipe containing water in which the infusion is used, in order to preserve the rest of the ingredients.*

Working with Surfactants, Preservatives and Emulsifiers

SURFACTANTS

In order to make wash-off products, you will need to use a surfactant (the term derives from 'surface active agent'), which is one of many different compounds that make up a detergent. Often foaming, surfactants work by breaking down the interface between water and grease or dirt. They hold the dirt and grease in suspension, thus easing their removal. Many wash products that are commonly available use petrochemical detergents, which can be harsh and drying on the skin. However, there are some more natural surfactants, derived from coconut, palm, starch and sugar, which are far preferable and these days easily obtainable from online suppliers of cosmetic ingredients.

We have used Plantapon LGC in several recipes: Seaweed and Herb Bath Essence (page 101); Hand and Body Wash with Rosemary, Mint and Basil (page 113); and Beer Shandy Shampoo with Lime Oil (page 126). This surfactant is from a natural, renewable source (it's derived from sugar and coconut oil) and is also biodegradable and mild in use. When combined with Lamesoft PO 65, a naturally derived moisture-restoring agent, it helps to thicken a product. The result is a gentle foaming base, adaptable for many uses.

Mix It Up

No heating is required if you're using Plantapon LGC: you can just mix it with Lamesoft PO 65, then with water and essential oils to make a finished product (you'll need to add a preservative if you plan to store the product; see right). You can also make an instant, water-based herbal infusion to add to the mix instead of plain water (see page 34). Fresh herbs from the garden, such as mint or lavender, are ideal. Alternatively, a tea infusion – such as camomile or green tea – or some aloe vera juice would work well.

The essential oils that you choose can reflect whether you want a refreshing, wake-up body wash (citrus or mint do the trick) or a relaxing, soothing foaming bath essence (with ingredients such as lavender, camomile or rose).

PRESERVATIVES

Preservatives are used in cosmetic products to stop the growth of bacteria, yeast, fungi and moulds. For a product to have any shelf life, it is necessary to preserve it.

When Do I Need to Use a Preservative?

- **Fresh recipes:** There are a number of fresh recipes in the book that are intended to be made and used immediately, or kept in the fridge for just a few days; these are mostly quick face masks. See, for example, the Cooling Gelatine Mask with Chlorella and Gotu Kola (page 83). For these recipes, no preservative is required.

- **Water-free (anhydrous) products:** If a product contains no water, or if it is purely an oil blend, then a preservative is not usually required, since it is water that forms a breeding ground for potentially dangerous bacteria and other microorganisms.

- **Powders:** Certain natural powders, although appearing to be water-free, will need to be sterilized to destroy any microbes; see, for example, the clay in the Face Mask with Clay and Camomile Tea (page 78). We recommend heating the powder in an oven at 100–120°C (212–248°F) and in most cases the addition of a preservative to the final product.

- **Products containing water:** Many of our recipes include water (including flower waters and aqueous plant extracts), and therefore list a preservative; we have chosen to use grapefruit seed extract (sometimes abbreviated as GSE), an entirely natural broad-spectrum antimicrobial that is safe, easy to use, widely available either from online suppliers or health-food stores, and has a long track record of efficacy in preserving cosmetic products. The usual dosage is 1 per cent, but in products with a pH of more than 7 (see page 40), it is advisable to increase the dosage. Having tested all our recipes using GSE when a preservative is required, we have increased the dosage in some cases to ensure the product is safe to use.

EMULSIFIERS

Emulsifiers are used to combine water and oil to allow them to mix and create a usable cosmetic product. Having tried and tested many emulsifiers, we have created our recipes using the following, because they are easy to use and readily available through online suppliers: Emulsifying Wax BP, a synthetic blend; Olivem 1000, a natural emulsifier derived from olive oil; and ESP Organic SafeEmuls SCA, a natural, organic blend of ingredients that creates particularly soft, mousse-like textures. It can be adapted by the addition of beeswax to achieve thicker creams and butters; see the White Nut Body Butter on page 109.

Recipes containing an emulsifier generally require some element of whisking or mixing to help the incompatible ingredients to combine. We usually suggest the use of a hand-held stick blender (or even a milk frother), because it's ideal for mixing very small quantities.

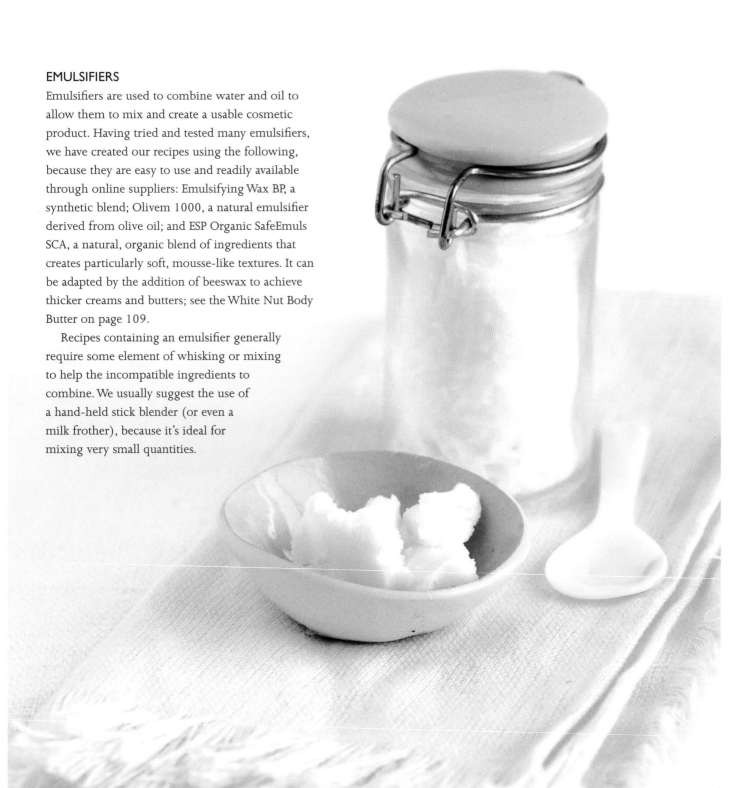

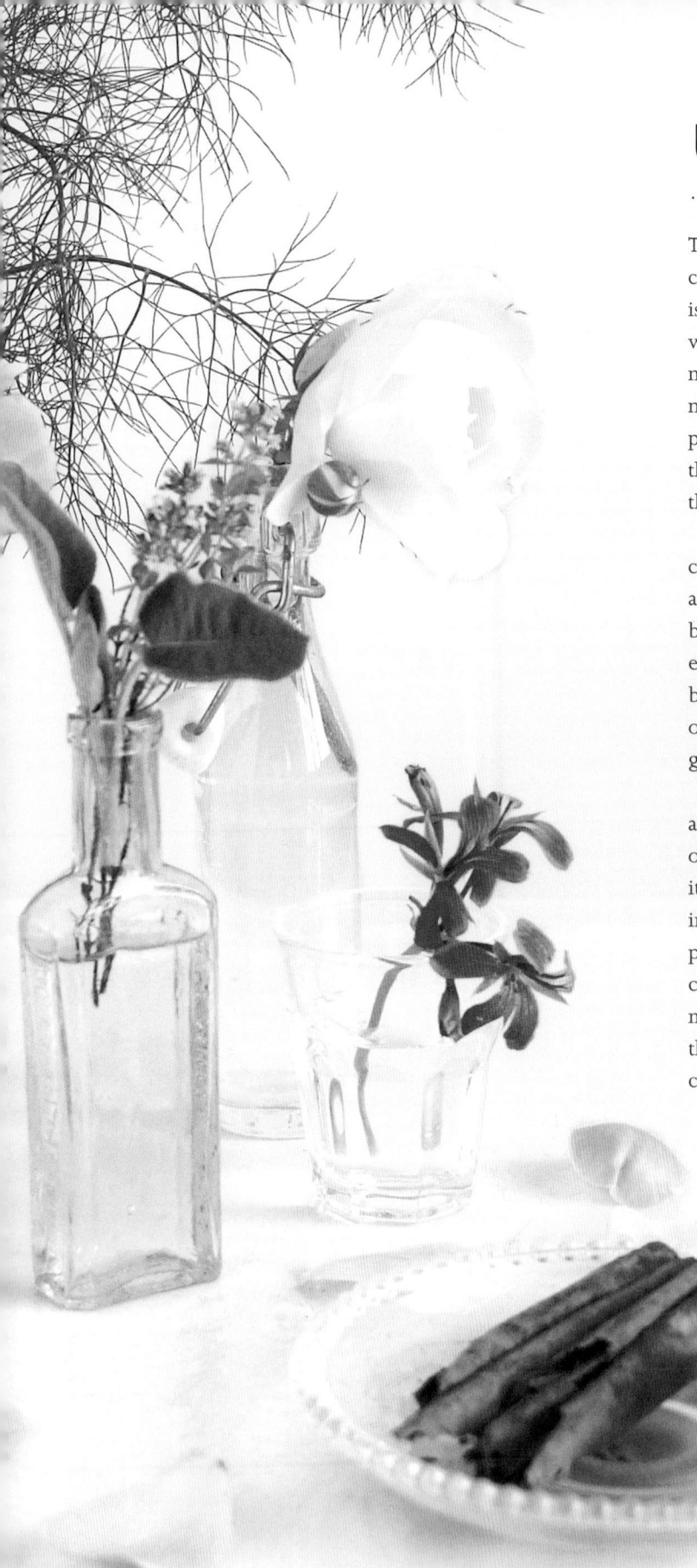

Using pH Strips

The pH of a substance is the measure of its acid or alkaline content in an aqueous/water-based solution. The pH scale is ranked from 0 to 14, with pH7, the natural acidity of water, being neutral. The further below 7 any value is, the more acidic it is; and, conversely, the higher above 7, the more alkaline. The pH of healthy skin is 5.5. Most cosmetic products are formulated to be close to the natural pH of the skin, so that they are gentle and work in harmony with the person using them.

As we have discussed on page 38, any product that contains water requires a preservative if it is to be stored and not used immediately. The recipes in this book have been chosen and tested to work with grapefruit seed extract; this preservative is effective over a broad pH range, but is most effectual when used in a product with a pH of less than 7. For this reason, we recommend the use of grapefruit seed extract when making these recipes.

Preservatives are effective within specific pH bands and therefore it is important when using any preservative other than grapefruit seed extract in a recipe to check its suitability and use it within the band for which it is intended. This information should be provided with the product when it is purchased. If you are in any doubt, check with the supplier. If the pH of the product does not fall within the efficacy range of the preservative, the product will be more susceptible to microbial contamination and therefore become unusable.

To Measure pH

You can measure the pH of a water-based cosmetic – prior to adding a preservative – by using pH test strips. These strips may be used in medicinal testing and home-brewing or even for monitoring the acidity/alkalinity of the water in fish tanks, and there are several types available. You can order packs online, or you might find them in a pet store or a shop selling home-brewing equipment. The strips have an infinite life, so one pack should last a long time.

On the test strips we use here, each strip has four indicator pads. On the strip container is a pH indicator chart that covers the complete pH range (0–14). For each pH value there is a corresponding colour sequence of four indicator squares. Once dipped in a product, each strip is compared against the squares on the chart; the matching colour sequence indicates the pH of the product.

ALTERING THE pH OF A PRODUCT

The addition of a few drops of lactic or citric acid solution reduces the pH of a product and is therefore useful for bringing it within the pH efficacy range of the preservative, if required. Recheck the pH each time you add more acid. For surfactant products combining Plantapon LGC and Lamesoft PO 65, lowering the pH of the product to about 5.5 can help to increase its thickness.

Note that it's unlikely you would need to raise the pH level of a product when following any of the recipes in this book.

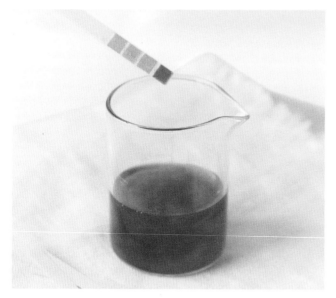

Step 1
For liquids and pourable gels, dip a test strip into the liquid for around 1 second, then remove. Don't get the strip too wet, or the indicator pads may peel off. For a cream, press the strip on the cream's surface for 5–10 seconds, then press the strip gently against a clean tissue for a few seconds to absorb excess product.

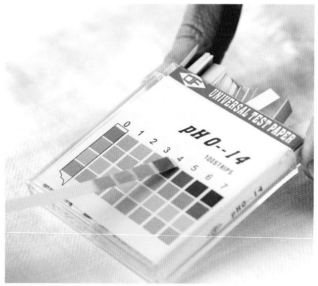

Step 2
Align the altered indicator pads on the strip with the matching coloured band on the indicator chart; this will tell you the pH number within a small but allowable margin that is sufficient for home use. For total accuracy, a pH meter is required, but the cost involved is almost certainly not necessary for home use.

Working with Dried Materials

We have many ingredients from which to choose when we're creating natural beauty recipes. As well as the natural oils, waxes or butters that help to create the right texture (in addition to their skincare properties, of course), there are some more unusual dried materials that can be incorporated for extra benefits.

FOR MASKS AND SCRUBS

Naturally absorbent and containing a concentrated source of minerals, clays often form the basis of face masks owing to their ability to draw out impurities from the skin; see, for example, the Face Mask with Clay and Camomile Tea on page 78. Clays, whether white or coloured, come in dried form. To ensure it's sterile, the clay powder needs to be spread on a baking tray (cookie sheet) and heated at a high temperature in an oven prior to use.

For body scrubs (see pages 104–107), it's necessary to use dried, quite solid, particulate ingredients in order to obtain an exfoliating action. In waterless products, these can be natural salts, such as sea, Himalayan or Dead Sea salt. Some seeds and grains, such as chia or poppy seeds,

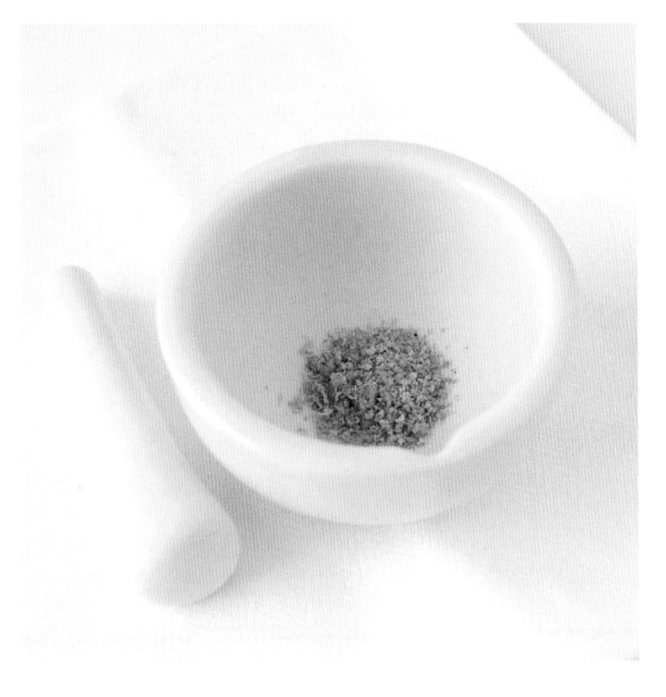

oat or rice, perform the same function, but are softer on the skin. They will, however, need to be heated in an oven for sterilization prior to use. Dried and ground seaweed are other good options to try. The salts have the advantage that they dissolve and easily rinse away.

In water-based products, hard nut-shell powders such as apricot, walnut and coconut work well. Sand and pumice make the hardest scrubs, and so are suitable for areas of tough skin, such as on the feet. They are generally compatible with both waterless and water-based recipes.

ADDING SUPPLEMENTS

We like to add vitamins, minerals and other supplements to many recipes, and most of these we have found in dry healthcare tablets or capsules. They provide a neat way in which to add a greater variety of concentrated and beneficial ingredients to skincare products.

- **Tablets** need to be ground to a fine powder using a pestle and mortar before being added to a recipe. For example, the enzyme from the exotic papaya fruit – which has the ability to exfoliate dead skin cells – is available as a tablet, and is a great addition to face scrubs, masks and cleansers, as in the Gentle Dispersing Face Scrub/Mask on page 77.
- **Capsules** must be broken open to dispense their contents, whether powder or liquid, for use. See, for example, the rhodiola and ginseng in the Eye Cream on page 86.

Vitamin C, available in both tablet form or as a loose powder, is extremely soluble in water, but quickly begins to lose its antioxidant potency in solution, so it is best added to waterless recipes, such as the Gentle Dispersing Face Scrub/Mask mentioned above, where, still fresh, its inclusion helps to brighten the skin.

Some of these powder materials can be difficult to incorporate into a recipe and may need to be added as a filtered oil- or glycerine-based botanical extract containing the infused beneficial properties of the plant or fruit, as in the Anti-Ageing Facial Oil on page 69.

Working with Sucragel Base

Makes 60ml (2fl oz)

INGREDIENTS
50ml (3½ tbsp) fractionated
  coconut oil
10ml (2 tsp) Sucragel CF

SPECIAL EQUIPMENT
plastic pipette
flat-bladed knife

Sucragel CF is a naturally derived ingredient, based on sugar, making it ideal for use in natural cosmetic recipes. It can be employed in different ways: for example, as an addition to an oil-and-water mix, where the Sucragel emulsifies the recipe, as in our Wipe-Off Cleansers (pages 50–52); or in a waterless gel, such as the Dispersing Eye Make-Up Remover Gel (page 59) and the Gentle Dispersing Face Scrub/Mask with Vitamin C, Manuka Honey and Papaya (page 77), where, with careful mixing, Sucragel is key in forming the gel structure and also provides cleansing, skin-softening properties.

The advantage of a waterless gel base is that ingredients such as vitamin C and papaya enzyme, which would degrade quickly in a water base, can be incorporated into products and retain their activity. The Eye Make-Up Remover Gel uses different oils to form a gel base that offers easy application in this concentrated format and yet is both gentle and highly effective. On rinsing with water, the dirt and make-up residue becomes emulsified and easily washes away.

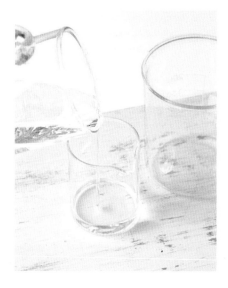

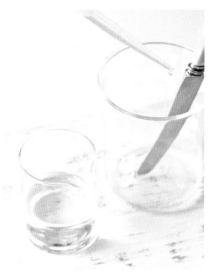

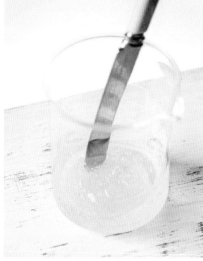

Step 1
Measure the fractionated coconut oil into a glass beaker or jug. In a second beaker, measure the Sucragel CF.

Step 2
Using a plastic pipette, gradually add the fractionated coconut oil to the Sucragel, a couple of drops at a time, while stirring with a flat-bladed knife (you can also use the reverse end of a teaspoon, but a knife works well as the gel thickens). At first the mixture will seem quite thin and oily, but as you add more oil, and stir it in briskly, the liquid will become increasingly gel-like.

Step 3
As the gel thickens, add the oil in greater quantity, increasing from a couple of drops to 2–3ml (½ tsp) at a time, and stirring until all the coconut oil is used up and a thick gel has developed. Owing to the air that has been incorporated, it will at first appear quite cloudy, but if you leave the finished gel for a few hours it will become entirely transparent.

Considering Storage and Safety

1. TAKE CARE WITH YOUR MATERIALS

- Always buy your ingredients from trusted sources and, once purchased, store them in airtight containers in a cool, dry place away from sunlight. Mark the container with the date of purchase. Before using materials, check they look good and don't smell 'off'; if in doubt, discard.
- For reasons of hygiene and safety, it is advisable to wear disposable vinyl gloves when measuring and handling raw materials, including essential oils.
- You should ideally use de-ionized or demineralized water in a recipe. Tap water can be used, but traces of metal salts are sometimes present that may cause products to discolour. Ensure water is boiled before use, to sterilize it.
- The materials we use must be properly treated so as to eliminate any microbes that could be harmful or spoil the finished product. Materials that contain water are particularly vulnerable to microbes, but remember also that materials that appear to be dry, such as flours or clays, can contain sufficient moisture to harbour moulds.
- We have carried out trials and micro-tests on each recipe, tweaking the method to ensure the finished product is free of microbes. It's vital that the methods are followed, especially where materials and phases require heating. We use the minimum '70°C (158°F) for 30 minutes' rule to kill off most undesirables. However, we also add preservative to water-based products to keep contamination at bay and extend their shelf life.

2. UNDERSTAND PRESERVATIVES

The preservative we have chosen to use is grapefruit seed extract, which is effective over a wide pH range (see pages 38 and 40). If you employ an alternative preservative, be sure to know its criteria for use; often there are tight restrictions as to the use level and the pH range at which preservatives are effective.

Waterless products, such as lip balms or body oils, generally do not require the addition of preservatives. However, we recommend adding preservative to powder products, as they can harbour microbes.

3. USE ESSENTIAL OILS CAREFULLY

We've already mentioned the potency of essential oils (see pages 24–25). Many neat essential oils can be potentially irritant, but the risks involved are very small if they are handled correctly. Ensure that the area you are working in is well ventilated. Take care not to get any oil in the eyes; if this should happen, rinse well with plenty of cold water.

4. STAY SAFE WITH EQUIPMENT AND STORAGE

- Use clean, sterilized tools and vessels when weighing, mixing and transferring products into containers. Fill containers to capacity; too much airspace aids oxidation.
- To avoid rancidity, store your finished products in a cool, dry place away from sunlight.
- Avoid dipping fingers into pots and leaving products without their lids, as these are ways by which microbes can be introduced and tax the preservative.
- Follow the shelf-life advice for each recipe, and check the smell, colour and appearance of your products before use.

5. KEEP A LOGBOOK

Keep a logbook with details of each batch of products you make: the date of purchase and source of each ingredient, the date of preparation, the phase temperatures achieved and the length of time the temperature was maintained. Note any variations you may make from the book recipes.

You may wish to check the pH of your water-based products (see page 41). If you see differences between batches of the same product, your logbook details may indicate the reason. We also suggest that you keep a small sample of each batch you make, for reference.

....

Remember! *The cosmetics industry is highly regulated; products undergo extensive trials and testing to ensure their safety and long shelf life. It's important to understand that the recipes in this book are intended for the home crafter and not for selling on to the public.*

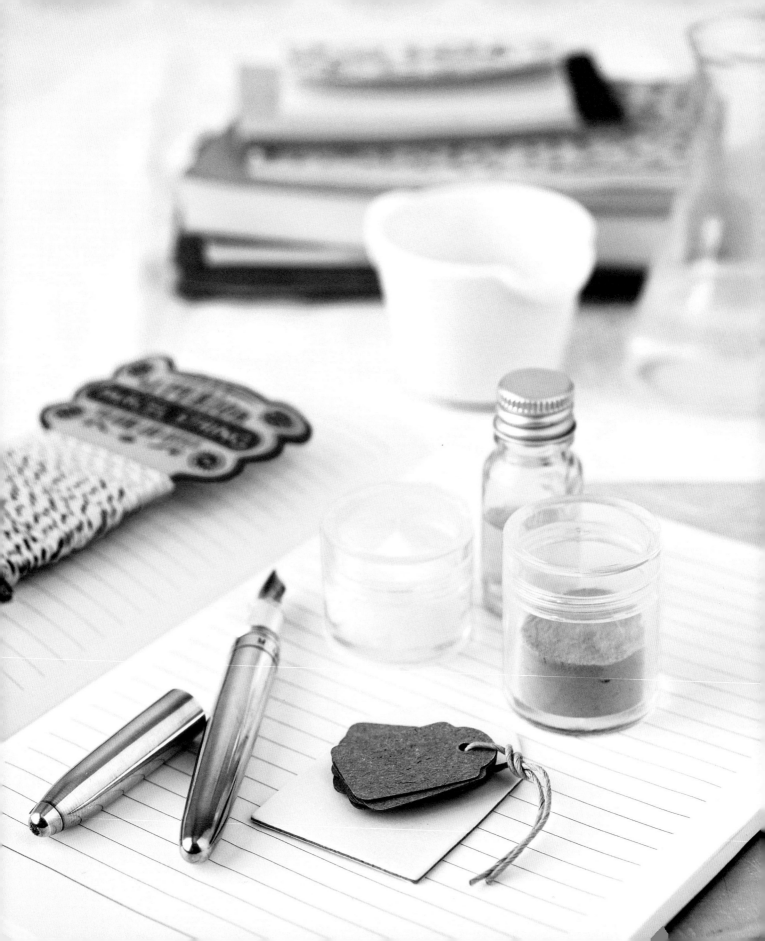

PRODUCT RECIPES

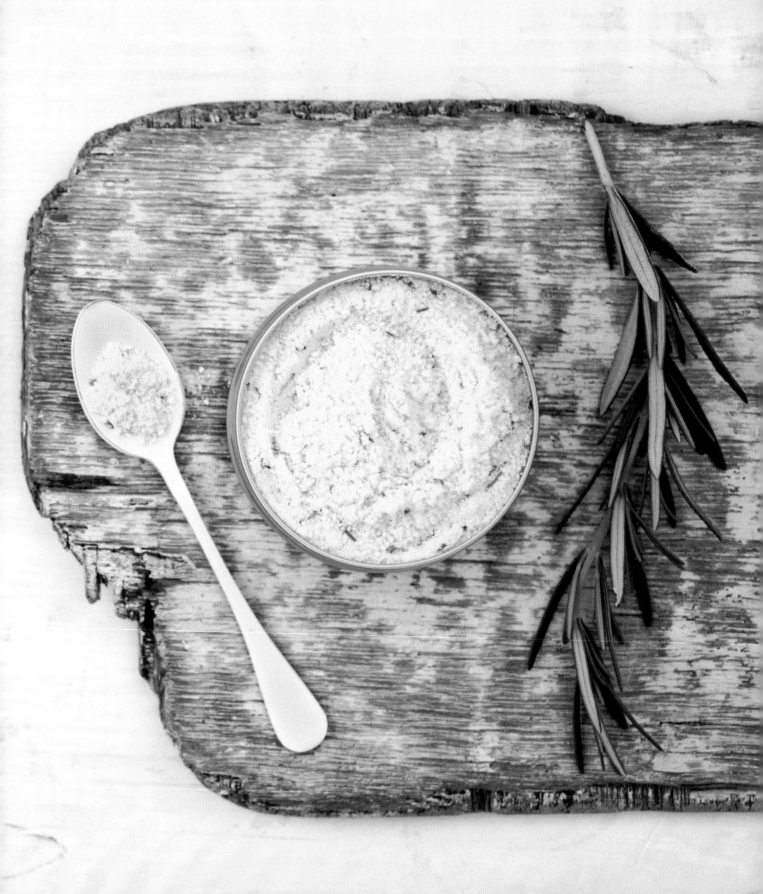

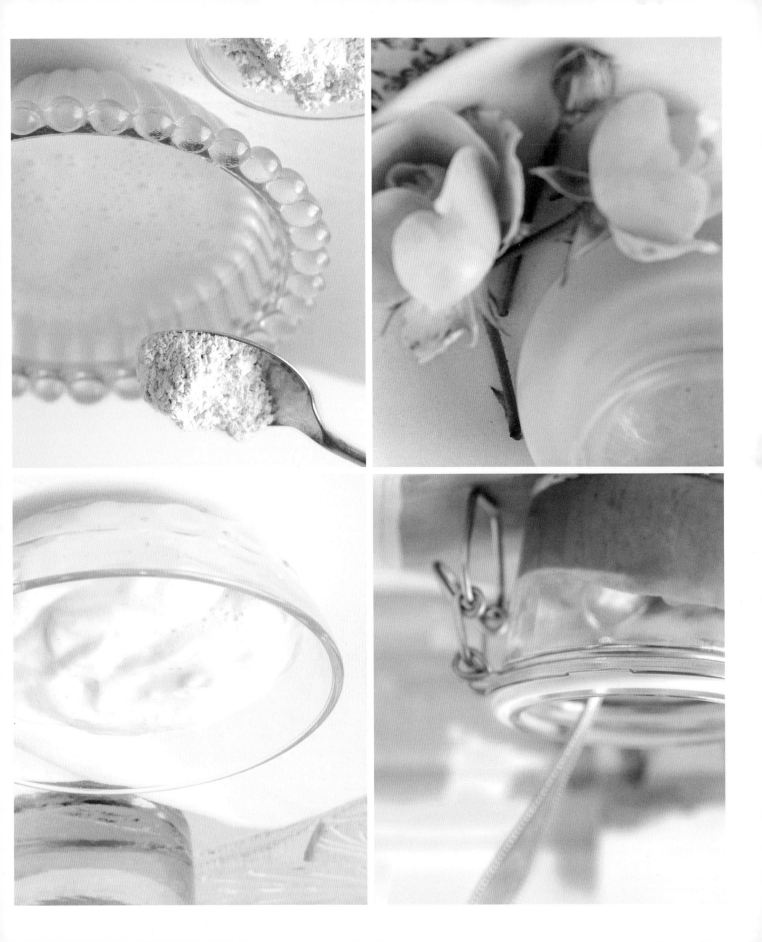

FACE

Wipe-Off Cleanser with Sucragel, Rose and Lavender *(for normal skin)*

Cleansing wipes have become really popular, but some can dry out the skin, and it is, in fact, very easy to create your own tailor-made wipe-away cleanser, whatever your skin type. What's more, cotton wool pads are a much nicer and more environmentally friendly way of applying cleanser to your skin.

Makes approx. 100ml (3½fl oz)

INGREDIENTS
26ml (5¼ tsp) rose water
40ml (2¾ tbsp) spring water
13ml (2½ tsp) Sucragel CF
20ml (4 tsp) fractionated
    coconut oil
5 drops lavender essential oil
40 drops grapefruit seed
    extract (as a preservative)

SPECIAL EQUIPMENT
thermometer

SAFE STORAGE
Store in a cool, dry place away from sunlight. Keeps for up to 3 months.

HOW TO APPLY
Shake well to mix, then pour a small amount on to a cotton wool pad and wipe gently across the face to remove make-up. No need to rinse. Follow with a toner appropriate to your skin type (see pages 60–65).

Alternatively, massage the cleanser into the skin to loosen make-up, and remove with a warm, damp facecloth.

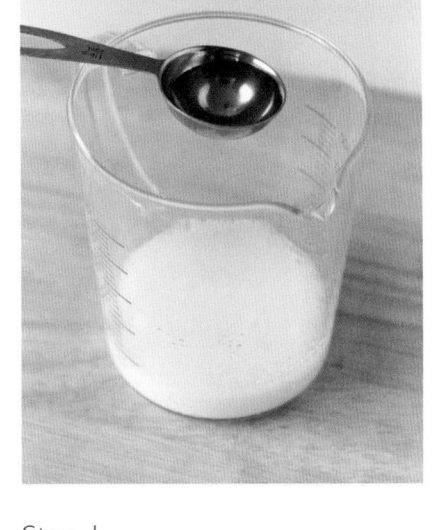

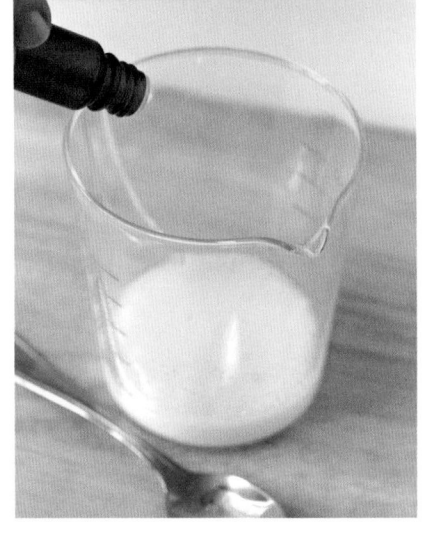

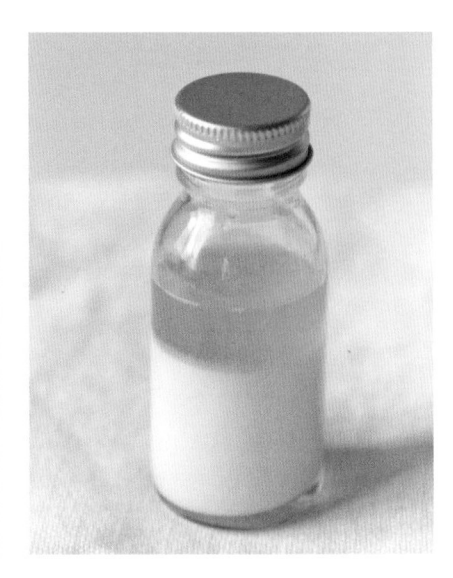

Step 1
Measure the rose water, spring water, Sucragel CF and fractionated coconut oil into a heatproof jug. Place the jug in a pan of simmering water and heat to 70–80°C (158–176°F).

Step 2
After 30 minutes, remove the jug from the heat and allow to cool to 30–40°C (86–104°F). Add the lavender oil and preservative, and stir with a stainless steel teaspoon to mix.

Step 3
Pour the mixture into a sterilized bottle with a cap. Label with the date and ingredients used. The contents will separate, so you'll need to shake the bottle before use to fully disperse the ingredients.

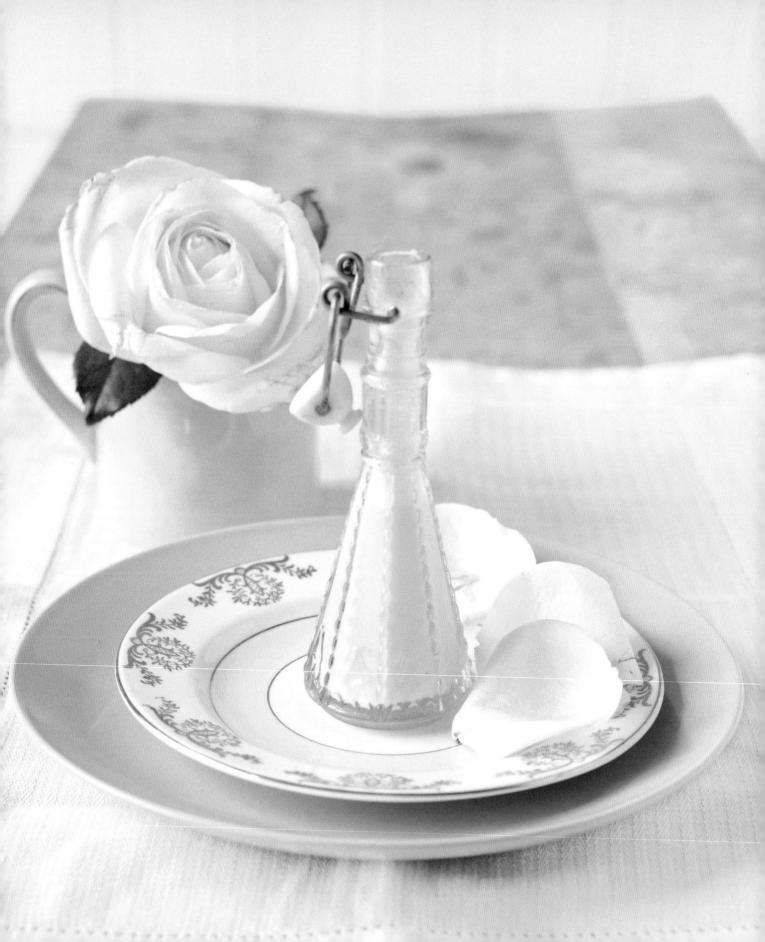

Wipe-Off Cleanser with Sucragel and Camomile (for sensitive skin)

This variation on the Wipe-Off Cleanser for normal skin has been adapted for sensitive skin, which is more susceptible to irritation from fragrances and some of the more active cosmetic ingredients. The addition of camomile essential oil here is particularly suited to sensitive skin, as it is traditionally used to relieve inflammation and calm troubled skin. Camomile essential oil is frequently sold diluted or blended in a carrier oil, such as sweet almond or jojoba.

Makes approx. 100ml (3½fl oz)

INGREDIENTS
66ml (4½ tbsp) rose water
20ml (4 tsp) rice bran oil
13ml (2½ tsp) Sucragel CF
5 drops camomile essential oil in dilution
20 drops grapefruit seed extract (as a preservative)

Measure all the ingredients except the essential oil and preservative into a heatproof jug, and follow the method for the Wipe-Off Cleanser for normal skin (page 50), adding the camomile oil and preservative after heating. Stir to mix, then pour into a sterilized bottle with a cap. Label with the date and ingredients used.

SAFE STORAGE
Store in a cool, dry place away from sunlight. Keeps for up to 3 months.

HOW TO APPLY
See the Wipe-Off Cleanser with Sucragel, Rose and Lavender on page 50.

Wipe-Off Cleanser with Sucragel and Thyme (for problem skin)

Problem skin has a tendency towards breakouts on account of blocked pores, but excessive cleansing may not be the answer. This variation on the Wipe-Off Cleanser for normal skin is a simple and effective option. It contains grapefruit and thyme essential oils, which have decongestant and astringent properties. Jojoba oil helps to moisturize, and orange flower water is both refreshing and delightfully scented.

Makes approx. 100ml (3½fl oz)

INGREDIENTS
66ml (4½ tbsp) orange flower water
20ml (4 tsp) jojoba oil
13ml (2½ tsp) Sucragel CF
2 drops thyme essential oil
3 drops grapefruit essential oil
40 drops grapefruit seed extract (as a preservative)

Measure all the ingredients except the essential oils and preservative into a heatproof jug, and follow the method for the Wipe-Off Cleanser for normal skin (page 50), adding the essential oils and preservative after heating. Stir to mix, then pour into a sterilized bottle with a cap. Label with the date and ingredients used.

SAFE STORAGE
Store in a cool, dry place away from sunlight. Keeps for up to 3 months.

HOW TO APPLY
See the Wipe-Off Cleanser with Sucragel, Rose and Lavender on page 50.

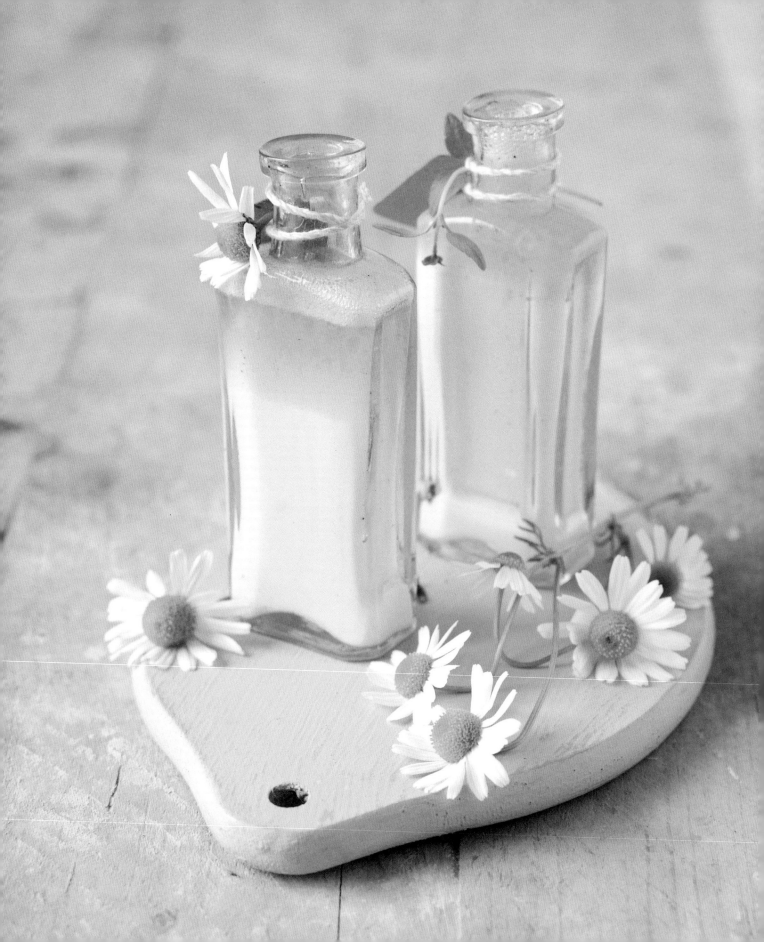

Japanese Gentle Exfoliating Cleansing Powder

This cleansing powder has a gentle exfoliating and skin-brightening action owing to the blend of rice or oat bran and kaolin. Vitamin C has antioxidant properties and helps to even the skin tone. Green tea and soluble aspirin soothe the skin, while Sucragel CF enables easy rinsing. The recipe will provide sufficient cleanser for several weeks' use, and is a great way to use your own flowers from the garden.

Makes approx. 60g (2oz)

INGREDIENTS
1 soluble aspirin tablet (300mg)
1 vitamin C tablet (1000mg or
   equivalent in powder)
2g (½ tsp) green tea (ideally
   loose leaf, not tea bags)
28g (1oz) kaolin (white clay)
28g (1oz) rice bran or
   oat bran
optional: 2 tsp dried calendula
   (marigold) petals (see page 20
   for drying instructions)
optional: 1 tsp dried lavender
   flowers
2ml (½ tsp) Sucragel CF
3 drops lavender essential oil

SPECIAL EQUIPMENT
small pestle and mortar
baking tray (cookie sheet)
coffee grinder

SAFE STORAGE
*Store in a cool, dry place away from
sunlight. Keeps for up to 3 months.*

HOW TO APPLY
*Mix a teaspoonful of powder with warm
water in the palm and massage into the
skin, avoiding the eyes. Rinse with a cloth.*

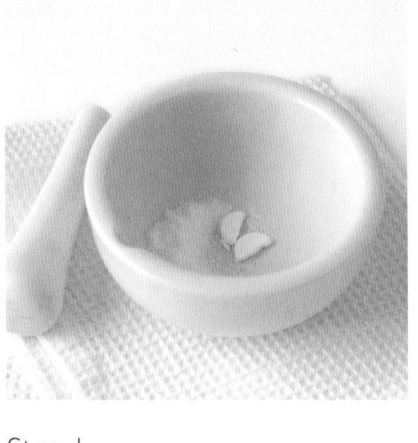

Step 1
Using a pestle and mortar, roughly crush the aspirin and the vitamin C tablet or powder, ensuring there are no large lumps left in the mixture.

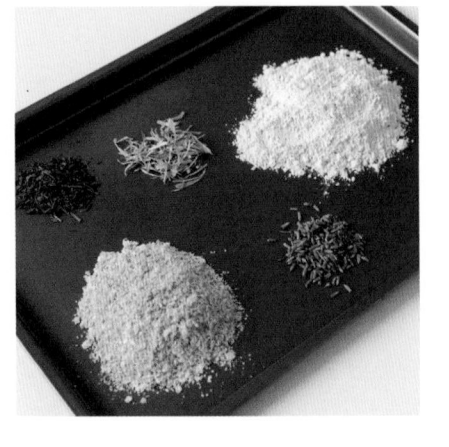

Step 2
Weigh the green tea, kaolin, rice (or oat) bran and flower petals (if using) on to a baking tray (cookie sheet). Place in an oven heated to 100°C (212°F) for 30 minutes.

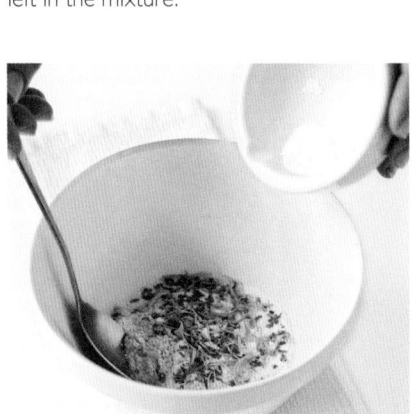

Step 3
Remove the tray from the oven and allow to cool. Place the contents in a bowl and add the crushed aspirin and vitamin C. Blitz briefly in a coffee grinder.

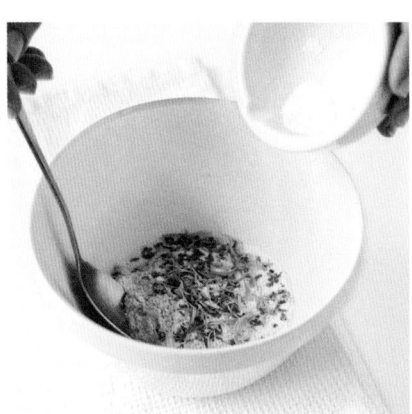

Step 4
Return the powder to the bowl and add the Sucragel CF and lavender oil. Stir, then pour into a sterilized, airtight jar. Label with the date and ingredients used.

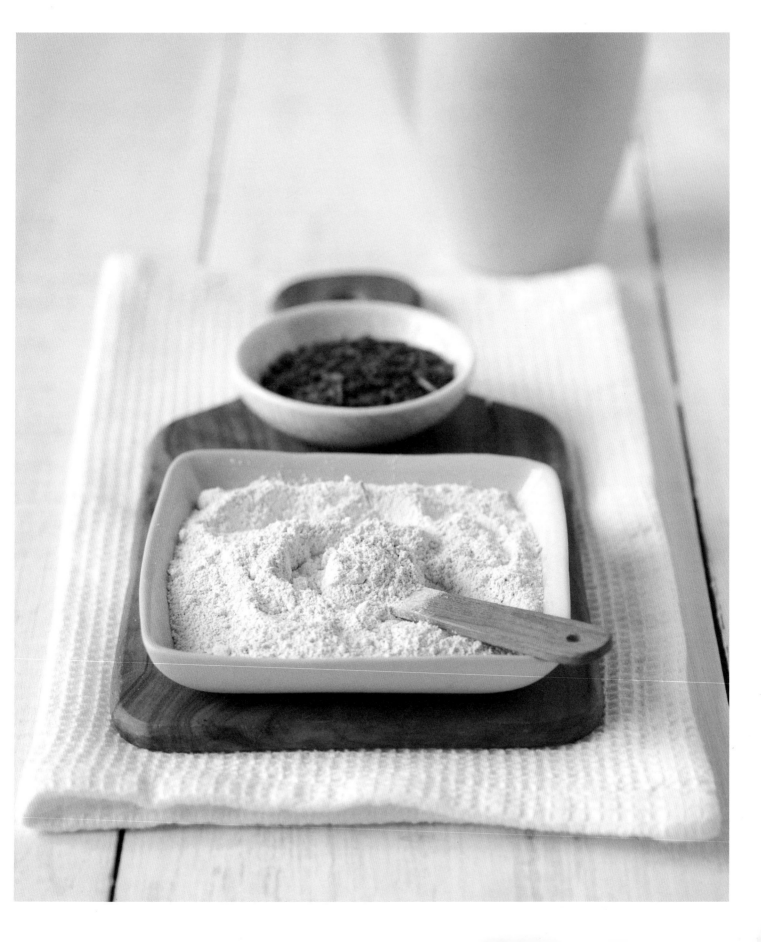

Eye Make-Up Cleansing Balm with Evening Primrose and Coconut Oil

An eye make-up remover should be both effective and sufficiently gentle to avoid rubbing and dragging the delicate skin around the eyes. Achieving this balance is all-important in creating the perfect recipe that lifts mascara, eye shadow and liner. This oil-based dispersing balm will gently but proficiently remove eye make-up, even some waterproof types. It is fragrance-free and soothing for use around the eye area. There is no water in the formulation, so there's no need for a preservative.

Makes approx. 100ml (3½fl oz)

INGREDIENTS
16g (½ oz) Emulsifying Wax BP
81ml (5½ tbsp) fractionated
   coconut oil
3ml (½ tsp) evening primrose oil

SPECIAL EQUIPMENT
thermometer

SAFE STORAGE
Store in a cool, dry place away from sunlight. Keeps for up to 3 months.

HOW TO APPLY
Dab or dispense a small amount on to a damp cotton wool pad and wipe gently around the eyes to remove make-up. No need to rinse.

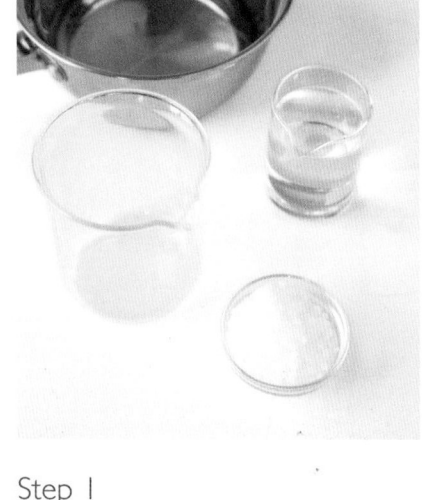

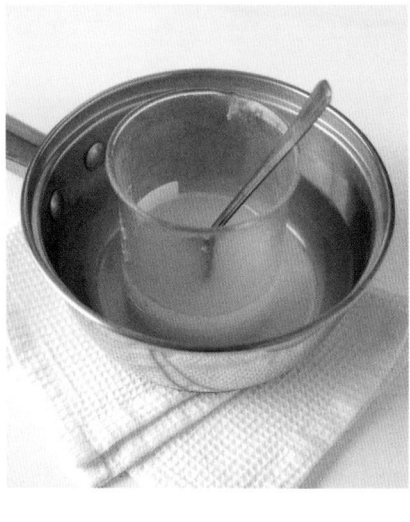

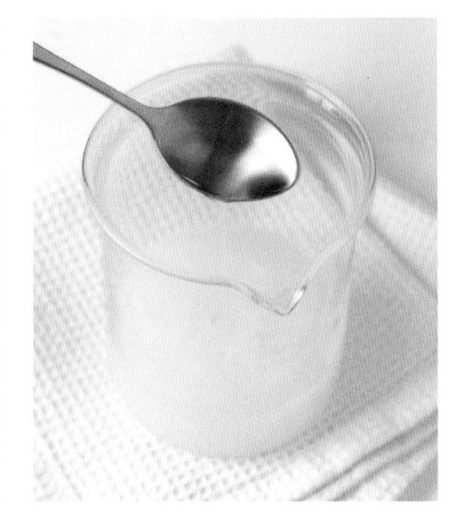

Step 1
Measure the Emulsifying Wax BP – which takes the form of small white waxy pellets – and fractionated coconut oil into a heatproof jug. Place the jug in a stainless steel pan of simmering water.

Step 2
Heat the jug, stirring with a stainless steel spoon to dissolve the Emulsifying Wax into the oil. Once it is dissolved, remove from the heat and allow to cool to 30–40°C (86–104°F).

Step 3
Add the evening primrose oil and stir to mix. Pour into a sterilized, airtight jar (or you can use a bottle with a pump dispenser if you prefer). Label with the date and ingredients used.

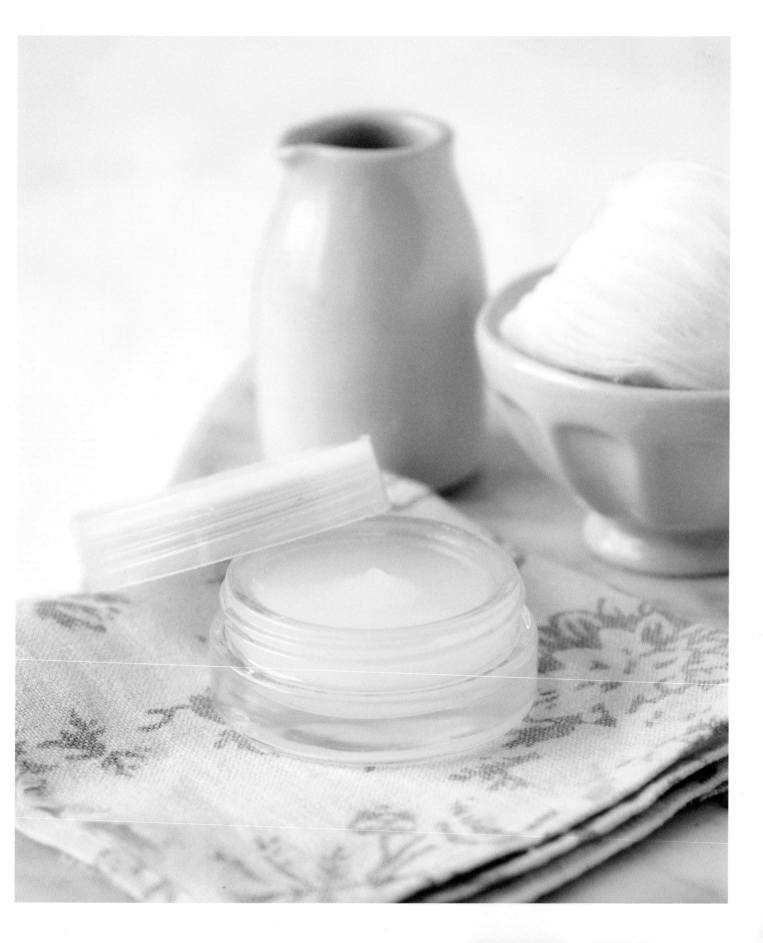

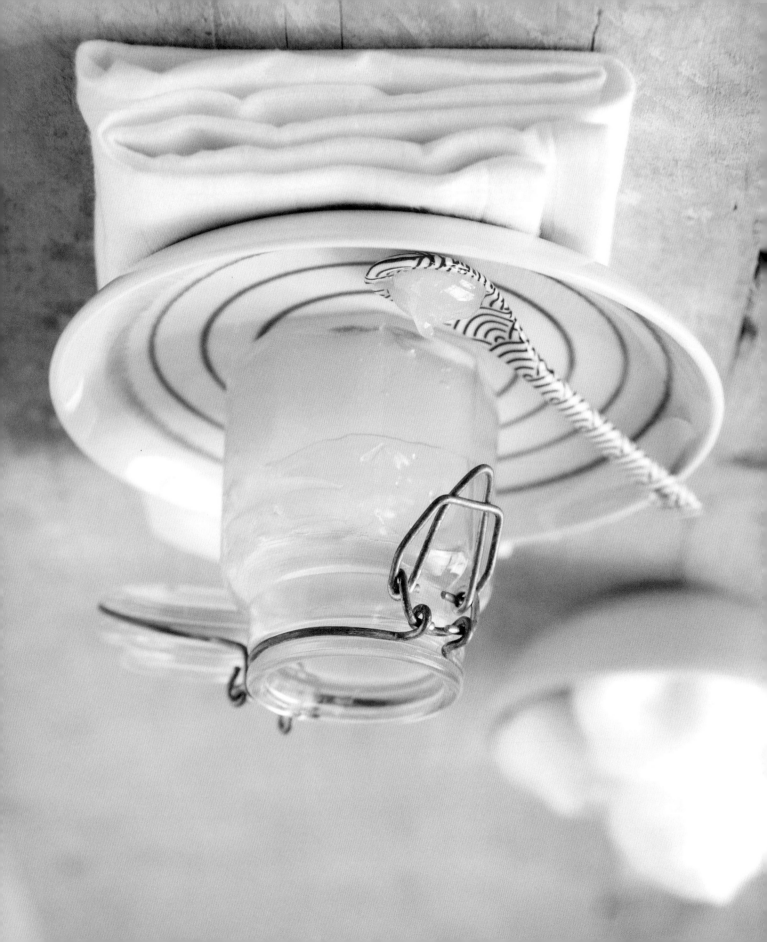

Dispersing Eye Make-Up Remover Gel

Here we've adapted the Sucragel base on page 43 to include a green tea glycerine infusion and nourishing oils that are beneficial to the delicate eye area. The resulting waterless, fragrance-free gentle cleansing gel is efficient at removing most eye make-up. The glycerine turns the original transparent base into an opaque gel, while the unrefined avocado oil adds a hint of pale green.

Makes approx. 60ml (2fl oz)

INGREDIENTS
38ml (2½ tbsp) grapeseed oil
2ml (½ tsp) rosehip oil
2ml (½ tsp) unrefined avocado oil
5ml (1 tsp) evening primrose oil
10ml (2 tsp) Sucragel CF
2ml (½ tsp) green tea-infused
  glycerine (see page 37)
12 drops grapefruit seed extract
  (as a preservative)

SPECIAL EQUIPMENT
plastic pipette
flat-bladed knife

SAFE STORAGE
Store in a cool, dry place away from sunlight. Keeps for up to 3 months.

HOW TO APPLY
Pour a small amount on to a damp cotton wool pad and wipe gently around the eyes to loosen make-up. Avoid pulling or stretching the skin around the eye area. Rinse with warm water, using damp cotton wool pads to wipe away any residue.

Tip!
The gel can also be used to remove face make-up and lipstick. It leaves the skin feeling amazingly soft!

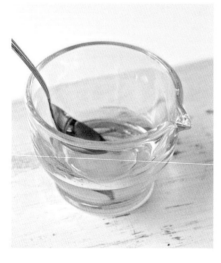

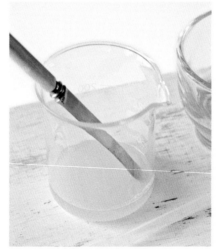

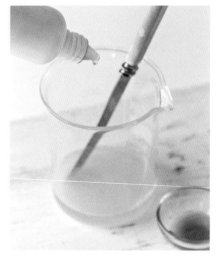

Step 1
Measure the grapeseed, rosehip, unrefined avocado and evening primrose oils into a beaker or jug, and stir together gently with a stainless steel teaspoon.

Step 2
Measure the Sucragel CF into a second beaker or jug and, using a plastic pipette, add the mixed oils, following the directions on page 43. Stir with a flat-bladed knife.

Step 3
Once gel-like, stir in the glycerine infusion and preservative. Pour into a sterilized bottle with a cap or a small airtight jar. Label with the date and ingredients used.

Skin-Brightening Tropical Toner with Coconut Water, Papaya and Ylang-Ylang

This exotic-sounding toner is made by using the basic method of mixing water, witch hazel and glycerine with essential oils. Inspired by the fruits and flowers of tropical islands, it also contains vitamin-rich papaya enzyme to help brighten the skin, as well as hydrating coconut water.

Makes approx. 100ml (3½fl oz)

INGREDIENTS
1 papaya enzyme tablet (60mg)
4ml (¾ tsp) glycerine
10ml (2 tsp) distilled witch
　hazel BPC
40ml (2¾ tbsp) orange
　flower water
20ml (4 tsp) coconut water
25ml (5 tsp) spring water
5 drops ylang-ylang essential oil
40 drops grapefruit seed extract
　(as a preservative)

SPECIAL EQUIPMENT
small pestle and mortar
thermometer
coffee filter paper
funnel (to hold the filter paper)
spray bottle with cap

SAFE STORAGE
Store in a cool, dry place away from sunlight. Keeps for up to 3 months.

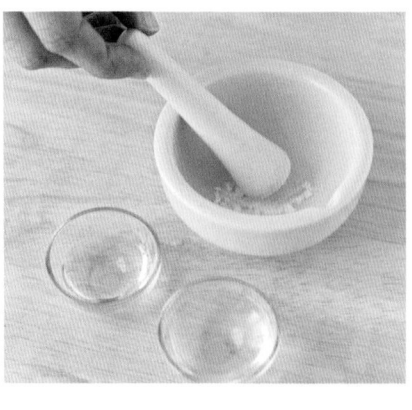

Step 1
Using a pestle and mortar, crush the papaya enzyme tablet; add the glycerine and mix thoroughly. Then add the witch hazel and stir to incorporate.

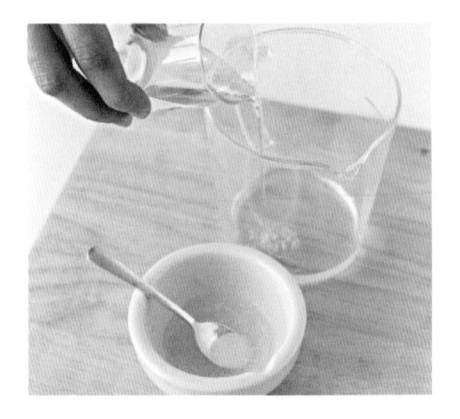

Step 2
Measure the orange flower, coconut and spring waters into a heatproof jug. Add the first mixture. Place in a pan of simmering water and heat to 70–80°C (158–176°F).

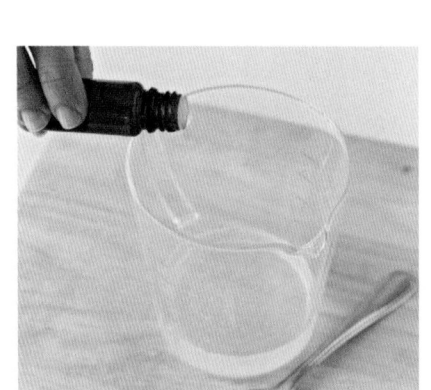

HOW TO APPLY
Spritz lightly on to thoroughly cleansed skin before applying moisturizer, to help hydrate and soothe.

Step 3
After 30 minutes, remove the jug from the heat and allow to cool to 30–40°C (86–104°F). Add the ylang-ylang oil and preservative, and stir to mix.

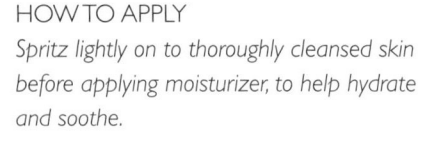

Step 4
Filter the mixture through a coffee filter paper to remove any solids. Pour into a sterilized bottle with a spray pump. Label with the date and ingredients used.

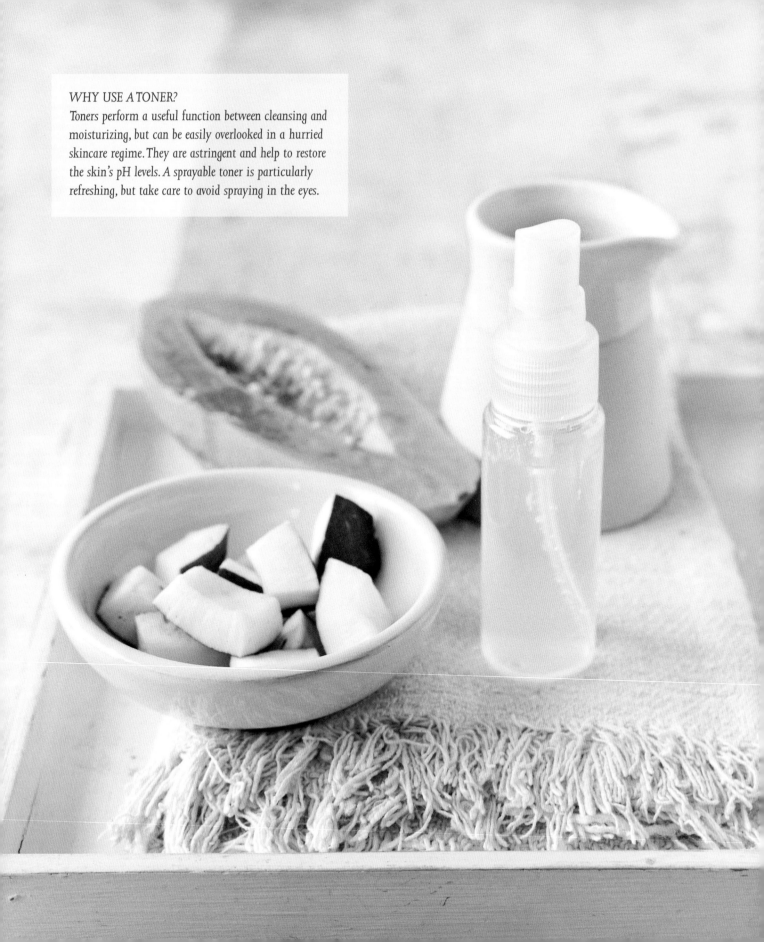

WHY USE A TONER?

Toners perform a useful function between cleansing and moisturizing, but can be easily overlooked in a hurried skincare regime. They are astringent and help to restore the skin's pH levels. A sprayable toner is particularly refreshing, but take care to avoid spraying in the eyes.

Toner with Juniper and Thyme (for problem skin)

This refreshing, clarifying toner is ideal for helping to balance problem skin. Thyme and juniper oils have traditionally been used to treat oily and acne-prone skin. Astringent witch hazel helps to keep pores clear. Thyme-infused glycerine is a useful and beneficial addition to this recipe, but plain glycerine is fine as an alternative.

Makes approx. 100ml (3½fl oz)

INGREDIENTS
90ml (6 tbsp) spring water
10ml (2 tsp) distilled witch hazel BPC
3ml (½ tsp) thyme-infused (see page 37)
  or plain glycerine
3 drops juniper essential oil
2 drops thyme essential oil
20 drops grapefruit seed extract (as a preservative)

Measure the spring water, witch hazel and glycerine infusion into a heatproof jug. Place the jug in a pan of simmering water and heat to 70–80°C (158–176°F). Maintain this temperature for 30 minutes. Remove from the heat and allow to cool to 30–40°C (86–104°F). Add the essential oils and preservative, pour into a sterilized spray bottle and shake to mix. Label with the date and ingredients used.

SAFE STORAGE
Store in a cool, dry place away from sunlight.
Keeps for up to 3 months.

HOW TO APPLY
Spritz lightly on to clean skin before applying moisturizer.

Refreshing, Sparkling Toner with Mint

Refresh and revive the skin with this zesty toner variation, combining oils of spearmint and peppermint with witch hazel, moisturizing glycerine and sparkling water. It's an excellent 'pick me up' to spray on your tired skin on a hot day. The sparkling water gives a natural 'fizz' to the toner, making it a true facial 'spritzer'.

Makes approx. 100ml (3½fl oz)

INGREDIENTS
90ml (6 tbsp) sparkling water
10ml (2 tsp) distilled witch hazel BPC
3ml (½ tsp) glycerine
3 drops spearmint essential oil
3 drops peppermint essential oil
20 drops grapefruit seed extract (as a preservative)

Measure the sparkling water, witch hazel and glycerine into a heatproof jug. Follow the method for the Toner with Juniper and Thyme (see left), adding the essential oils and preservative as a final step before pouring into a sterilized spray bottle and shaking to mix. Label with the date and ingredients used.

SAFE STORAGE
Store in a cool, dry place away from sunlight.
Keeps for up to 3 months.

HOW TO APPLY
Spritz lightly on to clean skin before applying moisturizer. This toner can also be applied during the day, even over make-up, to cool and revive the skin.

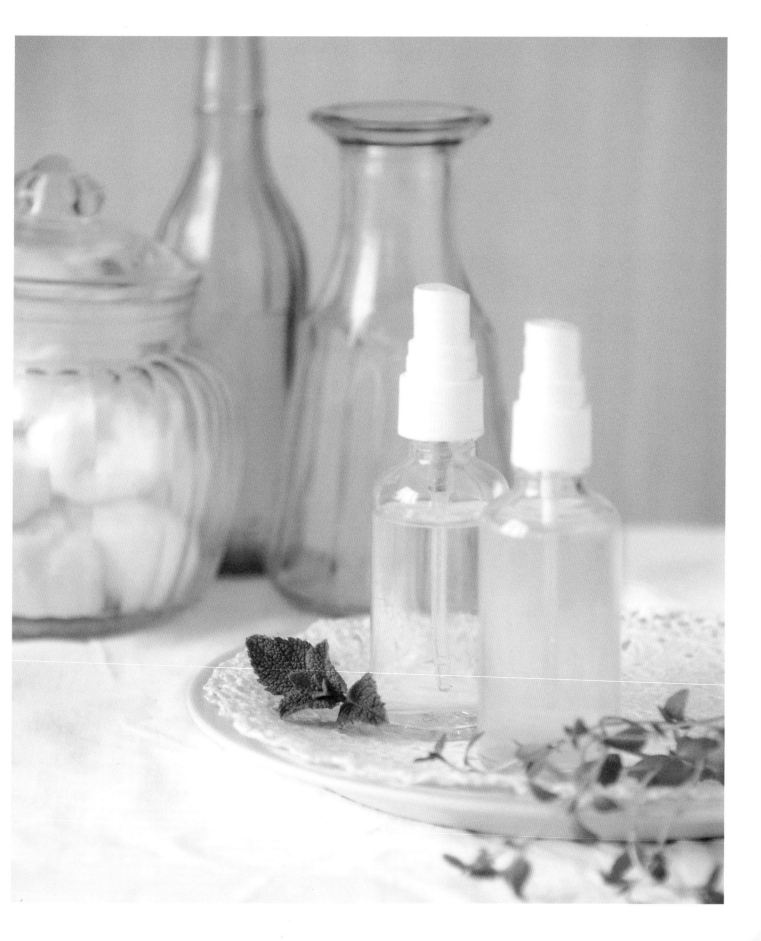

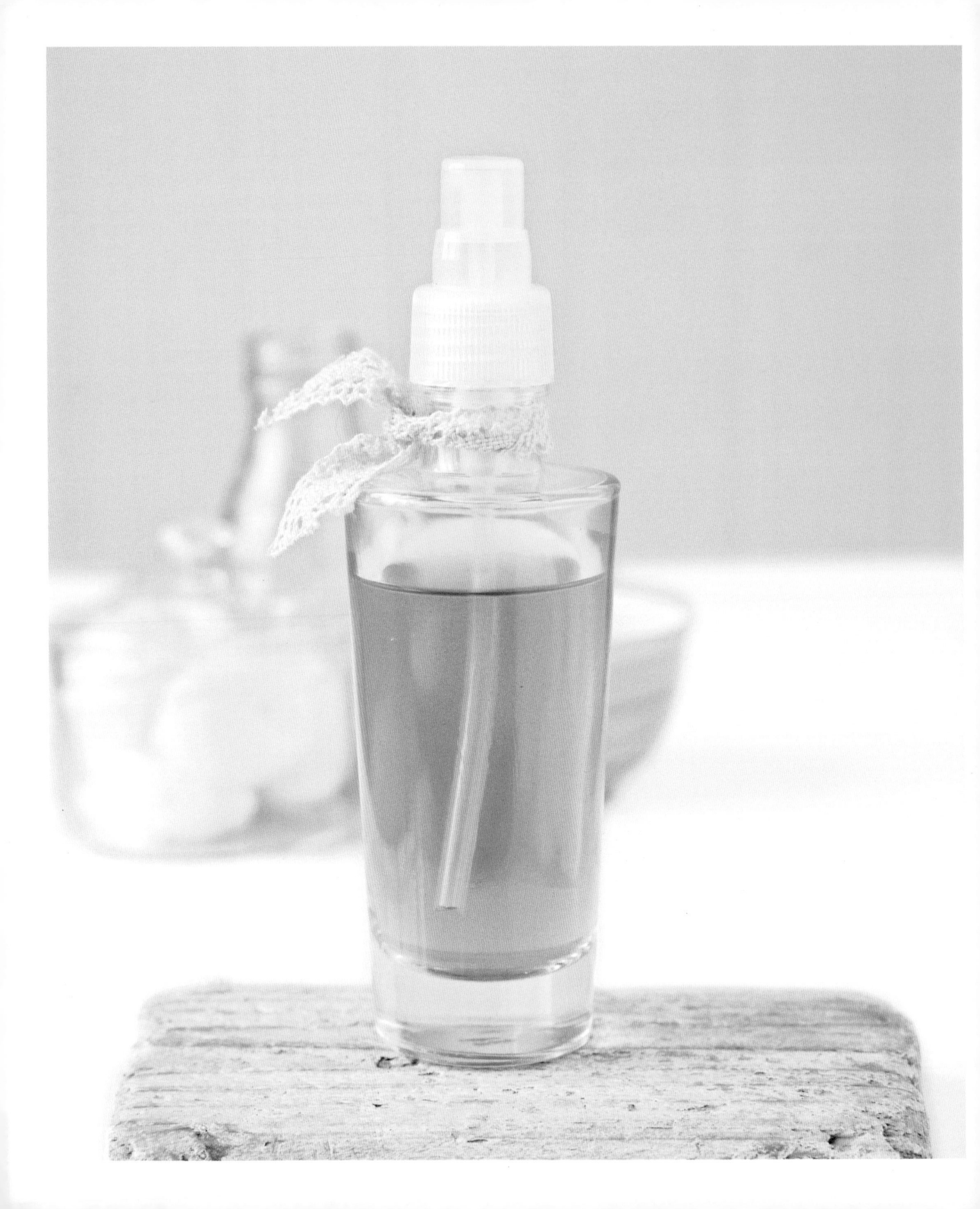

Antioxidant Toner with Acai Berry and Astragalus

Think pink with our hydrating toner, rich in antioxidants and vitamins contained in the acai berry juice and astragalus, a herb used in traditional Chinese medicine and infused here to extract the active components. Orange flower water lends a lovely light scent, making the toner wonderfully refreshing.

Makes approx. 100ml (3½fl oz)

INGREDIENTS
12ml (2½ tsp) acai berry juice
1 astragalus capsule (470mg)
10ml (2 tsp) distilled witch
 hazel BPC
77ml (5¼ tbsp) orange
 flower water
40 drops grapefruit seed extract
 (as a preservative)

SPECIAL EQUIPMENT
thermometer
coffee filter paper
funnel (to hold the filter paper)
spray bottle with cap

SAFE STORAGE
Store in a cool, dry place away from sunlight. Keeps for up to 3 months.

HOW TO APPLY
Spritz lightly on to clean skin before applying moisturizer, to help hydration. The citrusy, uplifting scent makes this a particularly good freshener to incorporate into your morning skincare routine.

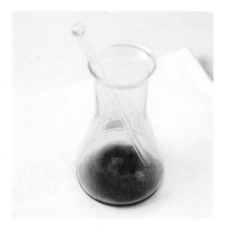

Step 1
Measure the acai berry juice into a heatproof jug or beaker. Break the astragalus capsule and carefully add the contents to the berry juice, stirring thoroughly to mix.

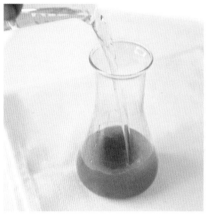

Step 2
Add the witch hazel and orange flower water to the jug. Place the jug in a pan of simmering water and heat to 70–80°C (158–176°F). After 30 minutes, remove from the heat.

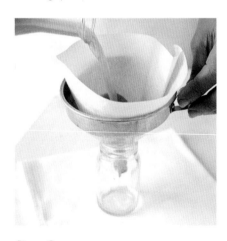

Step 3
Allow to cool to 35–40°C (95–104°F), add the preservative, and stir to mix. Once fully cooled, filter through a coffee filter paper before bottling.

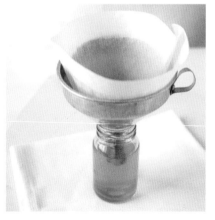

Step 4
The resulting toner should be light pink in colour and, once the astragalus is filtered, clear in appearance. Label with the date and ingredients used.

Fresh and Light Shea Butter Face Cream

Suitable for most skin types, this light face cream is simple to make. It's possibly the most popular recipe in the collection, and has been made time after time in our skincare classes. Some of the oils are adversely affected by heat, so they are added at the cooling stage. You can speed up the cooling process by placing the mixture in a large bowl half-filled with ice-cold water, as shown in Step 4.

Makes approx. 100ml (3½fl oz)

INGREDIENTS
Phase 1
3ml (½ tsp) glycerine
70ml (4¾ tbsp) orange
  flower water
10ml (2 tsp) sweet almond oil
7g (1½ tsp) Olivem 1000
5g (1 tsp) shea butter
3ml (½ tsp) vitamin E oil
  in dilution

Phase 2
2ml (½ tsp) evening primrose oil
5 drops neroli essential oil
  in dilution
20 drops grapefruit seed extract
  (as a preservative)

SPECIAL EQUIPMENT
thermometer
stick blender or milk frother

SAFE STORAGE
Store in a cool, dry place away from sunlight. Keeps for up to 3 months.

HOW TO APPLY
Apply to clean skin in the morning or at night. This cream is light enough to be used under make-up.

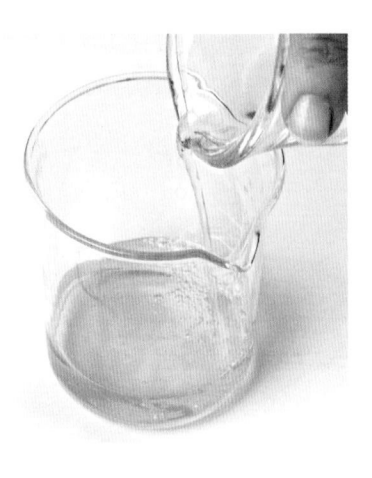

Step 1
Measure the glycerine, orange flower water, sweet almond oil, Olivem 1000, shea butter and vitamin E oil – all the Phase 1 ingredients – into a heatproof jug.

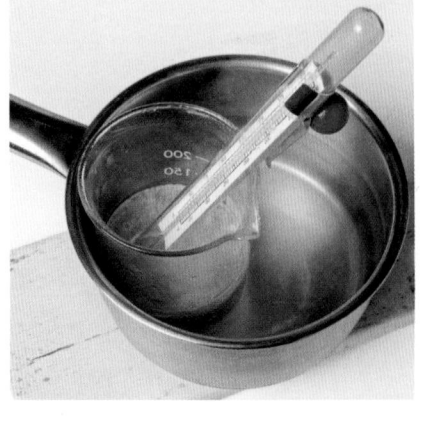

Step 2
Place the jug in a pan of simmering water and heat to 70–80°C (158–176°F), until the Olivem 1000 and shea butter have melted completely.

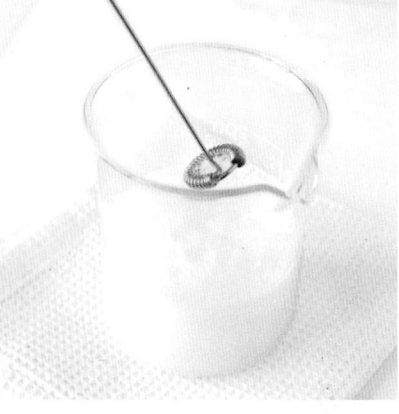

Step 3
Maintain the temperature for 30 minutes. Remove the jug from the heat. Whizz the mixture with a stick blender or milk frother.

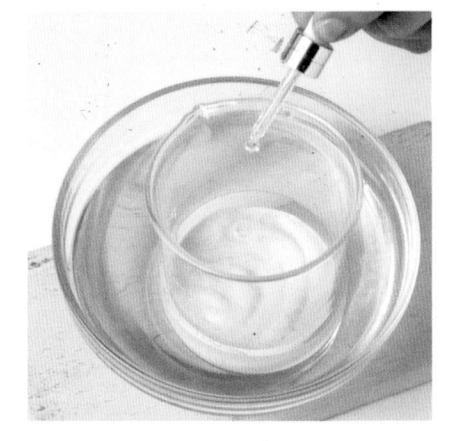

Step 4
Cool to 40°C (104°F) in a water bath, add the Phase 2 ingredients and stir. Pour into a sterilized, airtight jar. Label as usual.

Adaptation:
Shea Butter Night Cream

When you need a really nourishing night-time fix, try this rich cream. The jasmine essential oil gives it a thoroughly indulgent feel, while the organic emulsifier and the beeswax make it a very natural recipe.

Makes approx. 100ml (3½fl oz)

INGREDIENTS
5ml (1 tsp) glycerine
60ml (4 tbsp) rose water
10ml (2 tsp) grapeseed oil
10g (¼oz) shea butter
10g (¼oz) ESP Organic SafeEmuls SCA
4g (¾ tsp) beeswax white BP
6 drops jasmine essential oil in dilution
20 drops grapefruit seed extract (as a preservative)

Measure all the ingredients apart from the jasmine oil and preservative into a heatproof jug. Follow the method for the Fresh and Light Shea Butter Face Cream (opposite). After the mixture has cooled to 40°C (104°F), add the jasmine oil and preservative. Stir to mix thoroughly and pour into a sterilized, airtight jar. Label with the date and ingredients used.

SAFE STORAGE
Store in a cool, dry place away from sunlight.
Keeps for up to 3 months.

HOW TO APPLY
Apply to clean skin at night. Because the cream is slow to be absorbed, it can also be used as a massage lotion, applied with light, upward strokes. Although the finished recipe has a lotion-like texture, it is very protective, so it is also ideal for use in wintry weather.

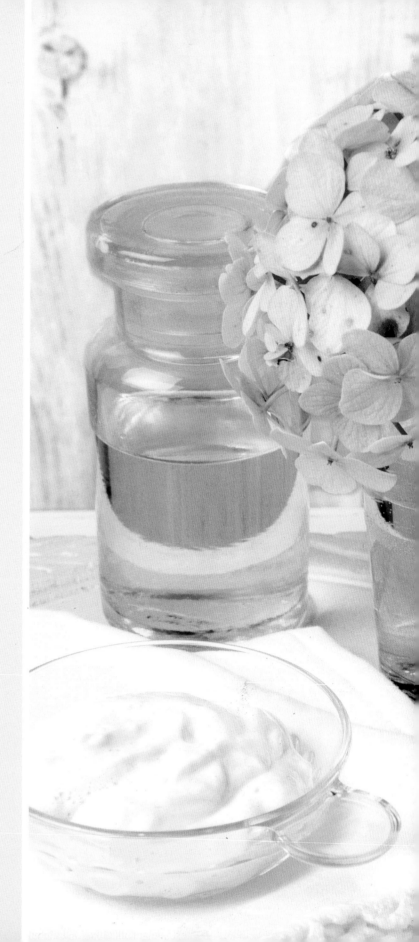

Nourishing Facial Oil

Makes approx. 50ml (1 ½fl oz)

INGREDIENTS
20ml (4 tsp) rice bran oil
10ml (2 tsp) vitamin E oil
 in dilution
7ml (1 ½ tsp) argan oil
13ml (2 ½ tsp) rosehip oil
2 drops geranium essential oil

SPECIAL EQUIPMENT
glass bottle with dropper

SAFE STORAGE
Store in a cool, dry place away from sunlight. Keeps for up to 6 months.

HOW TO APPLY
Using your fingertips, massage a small amount into clean skin with circular movements (see below). Apply at night.

MASSAGING YOUR FACE WITH OIL
Massage will not only help a facial oil to be absorbed but also relaxes the skin. Pour a small amount of oil into the palm of the hand and gently apply all over the face, avoiding the eyes. Begin at the chin, massaging with your fingertips using small circular movements. Massage either side of the mouth and nose, along the cheekbones and outwards to the temples. Apply gentle but firm pressure either side of the eyes and around the eyebrows to relieve any tension. Finally, using your palms, stroke the oil up the forehead to the hairline.

Facial oils are very popular these days, and this lovely light version is particularly easy to make. It is ideal for normal to dry skins, and a terrific treat for tired skin in winter. It will absorb into the skin surprisingly quickly and really doesn't feel greasy, as you might expect. It is best applied at bedtime. Alternatively, it also works well as a light massage oil to relax the face. Vitamin E oil, which promotes the healing and fading of scars, is usually available in dilution with a carrier oil, such as sweet almond oil.

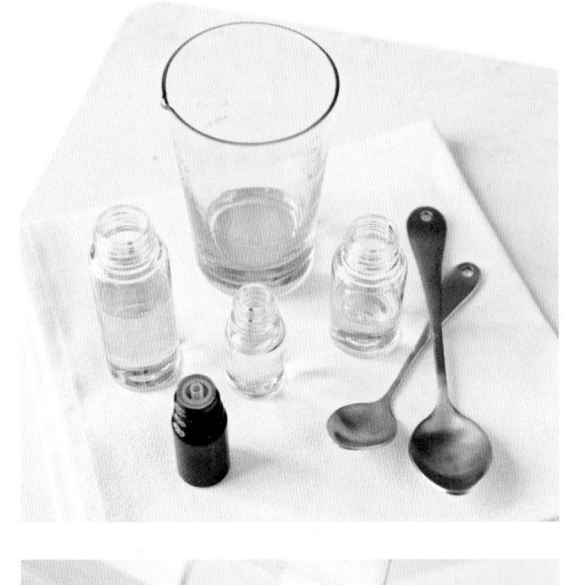

Step 1
The recipe will take only a few minutes to make, particularly if you use measuring spoons, which can be quicker than weighing ingredients. But before you get started, check that your oils are free of any rancid odours, as these will result in an unpleasant, 'off'-smelling final product. Simply measure all the ingredients into a glass jug or beaker.

Step 2
Stir with a stainless steel teaspoon to mix the oils and then pour into a sterilized, airtight glass bottle, ideally with a dropper, which will enable you to control the number of drops you dispense. Label with the date and ingredients used.

Anti-Ageing Facial Oil

Our alternative facial oil uses infused astragalus and coenzyme Q10 to give the skin a really powerful shot of restorative antioxidants.

Makes approx. 50ml (1½fl oz)

INGREDIENTS
1 coenzyme Q10 tablet (30mg)
1 astragalus capsule (470mg)
20ml (4 tsp) rice bran oil
10ml (2 tsp) vitamin E oil in dilution
5ml (1 tsp) refined avocado oil
15ml (3 tsp) rosehip oil
1 drop frankincense essential oil
2 drops jasmine essential oil in dilution
1 evening primrose oil capsule (500mg)

Crush the coenzyme Q10 tablet using a small pestle and mortar, and add the contents of the astragalus capsule. Infuse the astragalus and coenzyme Q10 in the rice bran oil and pour into a glass jug. Cover and then leave to infuse further overnight. Filter the infusion using a coffee filter paper and a funnel. Add the remaining ingredients and stir to mix. Pour into a sterilized, airtight glass bottle with a dropper. Label with the date and ingredients used.

SAFE STORAGE
Store in a cool, dry place away from sunlight.
Keeps for up to 6 months.

HOW TO APPLY
Using your fingertips, massage a small amount into clean skin with circular movements (see 'Massaging Your Face with Oil' opposite).

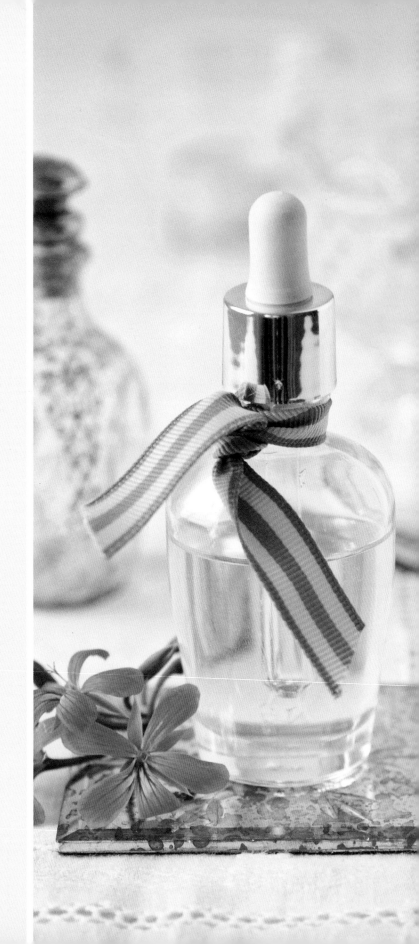

Face Lotion with Thyme and Grapefruit

(for problem skin)

Use this light lotion to hydrate, but not overload, oily and breakout-prone skin. Thyme is known for its antibacterial and antiseptic qualities. Sage is also antimicrobial, but if you prefer you can use plain glycerine instead of the sage infusion (see page 37). Grapefruit essential oil adds a delicious freshness.

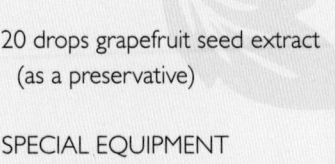
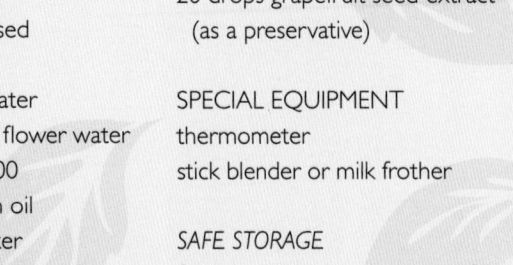
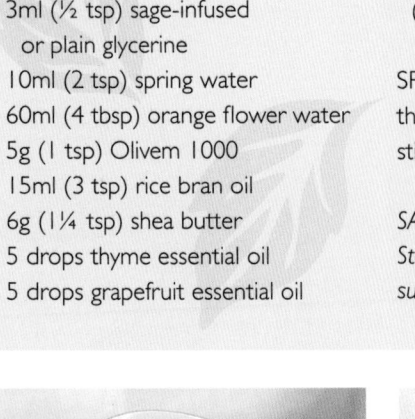

Makes approx. 100ml (3½fl oz)

INGREDIENTS
3ml (½ tsp) sage-infused
  or plain glycerine
10ml (2 tsp) spring water
60ml (4 tbsp) orange flower water
5g (1 tsp) Olivem 1000
15ml (3 tsp) rice bran oil
6g (1¼ tsp) shea butter
5 drops thyme essential oil
5 drops grapefruit essential oil

20 drops grapefruit seed extract
  (as a preservative)

SPECIAL EQUIPMENT
thermometer
stick blender or milk frother

SAFE STORAGE
Store in a cool, dry place away from sunlight. Keeps for up to 3 months.

HOW TO APPLY
Apply to clean skin in the morning or at night. The scent is particularly uplifting for daytime use. Owing to the combination of a natural emulsifier, Olivem 1000 (see page 39), with moisturizing shea butter and light rice bran oil, this lotion is light enough to be used under make-up. Wait a few minutes for the lotion to be properly absorbed before applying your cosmetic base.

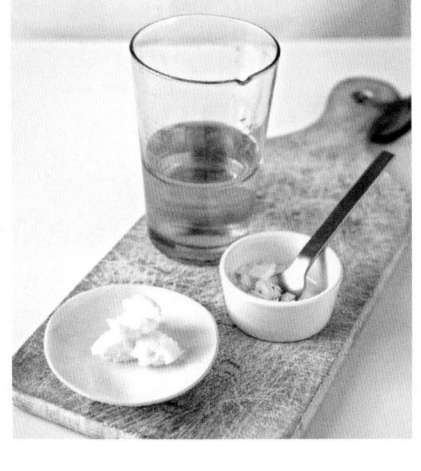

Step 1
Weigh all the ingredients except the essential oils and preservative into a heatproof jug. Place the jug in a pan of simmering water and heat to 70°C (158°F).

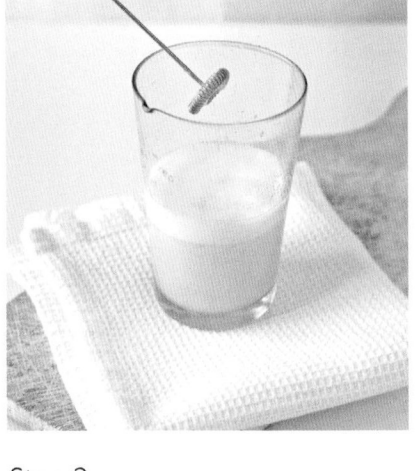

Step 2
Maintain the temperature for 30 minutes, then remove the jug from the heat and allow the contents to cool slightly. Whizz with a stick blender or milk frother to mix thoroughly.

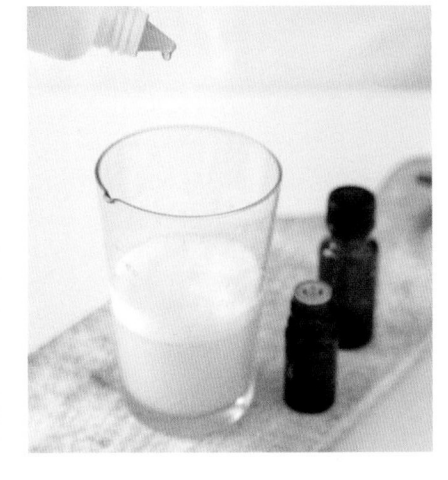

Step 3
Allow the mixture to de-aerate and cool to around 40°C (104°F), then add the essential oils and preservative. Pour into a sterilized bottle with a cap. Label with the date and ingredients used.

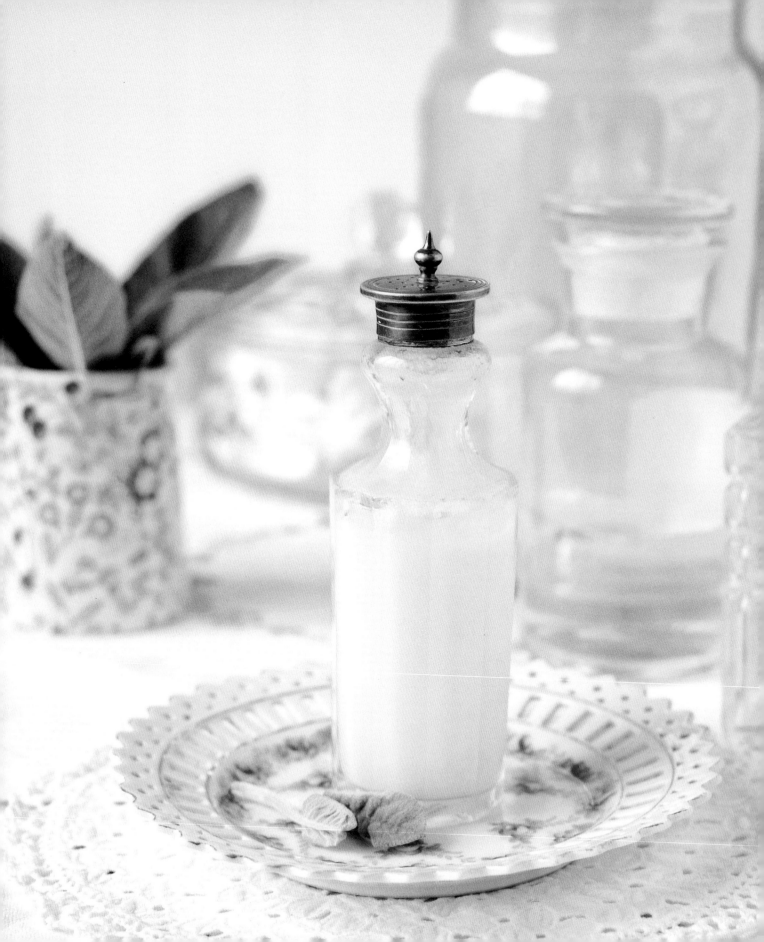

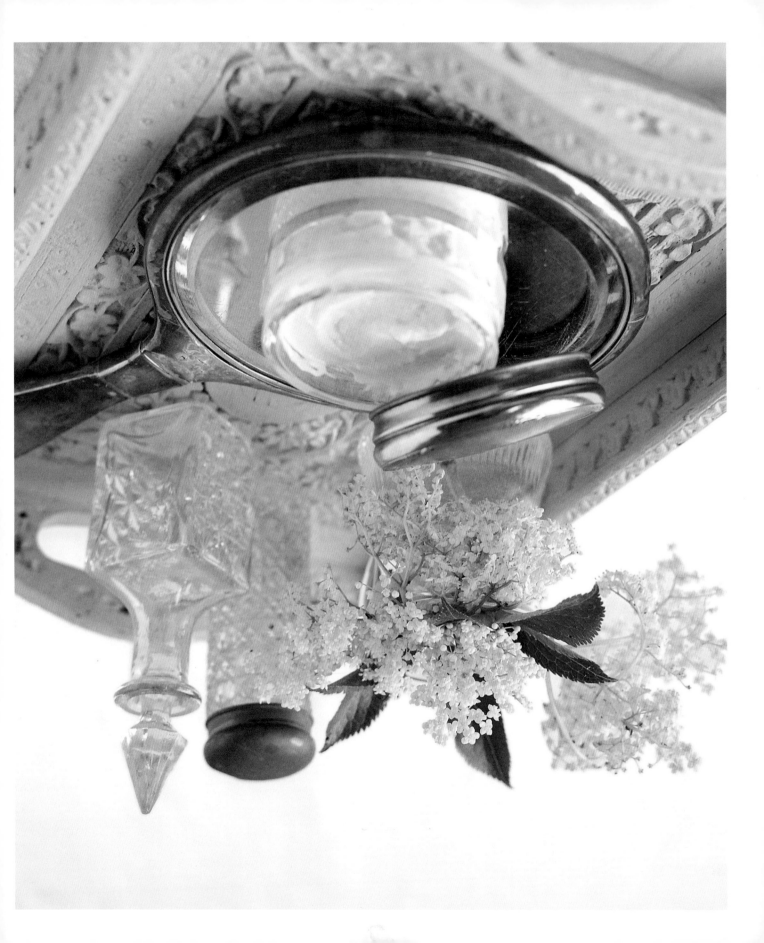

Anti-Pigmentation Night Cream

This protective cream contains elderflower-infused glycerine. Elderflowers have a long history of use as a skin-lightening ingredient; if they're not available, you can use a liquorice infusion instead. On account of its luxuriously rich texture, the cream is best applied as a restorative treat at bedtime.

Makes approx. 100ml (3½fl oz)

INGREDIENTS

Phase 1
52ml (3½ tbsp) rose water
5ml (1 tsp) elderflower- or
   liquorice-infused glycerine
14ml (2¾ tsp) rice bran oil
10g (¼oz) shea butter
7g (1½ tsp) Emulsifying Wax BP

Phase 2
10ml (2 tsp) rosehip oil
5 drops jasmine essential oil
   in dilution
5 drops frankincense
   essential oil
40 drops grapefruit seed extract
   (as a preservative)

SPECIAL EQUIPMENT
optional: glass rod
thermometer
stick blender or milk frother

SAFE STORAGE
*Store in a cool, dry place away
from sunlight. Keeps for up to
3 months.*

HOW TO APPLY
*Gently smooth a thin layer on to clean
skin at night.*

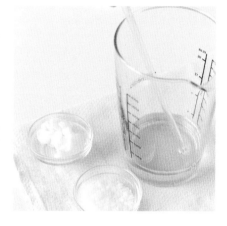

Step 1
Measure the Phase 1 ingredients into a heatproof jug and stir with a glass rod or stainless steel spoon to mix. (See page 37 for instructions on making an infusion.)

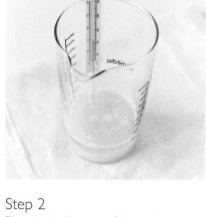

Step 2
Place the jug in a pan of simmering water and heat to 70°C (158°F). Maintain this temperature for 30 minutes, then remove from the heat.

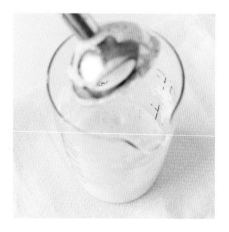

Step 3
Whizz the mixture with a stick blender or milk frother. Cool to around 40°C (104°F), but don't allow to set. Add all the Phase 2 ingredients, and stir to mix thoroughly.

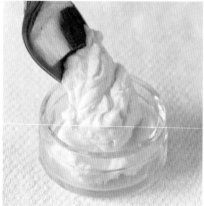

Step 4
Spoon into a sterilized, airtight jar and secure the lid once the mixture has cooled; the cream will be quite thick. Label with the date and ingredients used.

Intensive Anti-Ageing Night Cream with Astragalus and Five Oils

Packed full of anti-ageing oils and supplements, this cream is a winning formula at any time of the year, but particularly beneficial in winter. Owing to the number of ingredients and phases, it's a little more time-consuming than most recipes, but worth the effort!

Makes approx. 100ml (3½fl oz)

INGREDIENTS

Phase 1

1 resveratrol capsule (50mg)

4ml (¾ tsp) evening primrose oil

Phase 2

50ml (3½ tbsp) rose water

1 astralgalus capsule (470mg)

Phase 3

5ml (1 tsp) camomile-infused glycerine (see page 37)

12g (½oz) ESP Organic SafeEmuls SCA

2g (½ tsp) beeswax white BP

10ml (2 tsp) shea butter

3ml (½ tsp) refined avocado oil

3ml (½ tsp) wheatgerm oil

Phase 4

4ml (¾ tsp) rosehip oil

20 drops geranium essential oil

20 drops grapefruit seed extract (as a preservative)

SPECIAL EQUIPMENT

scissors

thermometer

stick blender or milk frother

SAFE STORAGE

Store in a cool, dry place away from sunlight. Keeps for up to 3 months.

HOW TO APPLY

Apply a thin layer to clean skin at night.

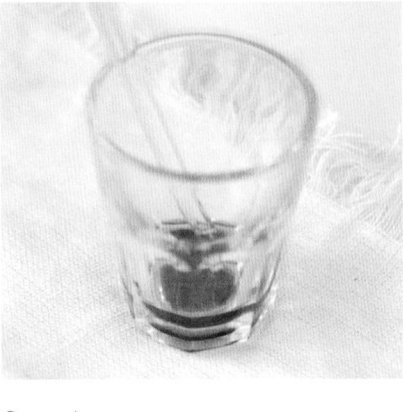

Step 1

Snip the resveratrol capsule with sharp scissors and squeeze the contents into a small beaker or glass. Add the evening primrose oil and stir to mix fully.

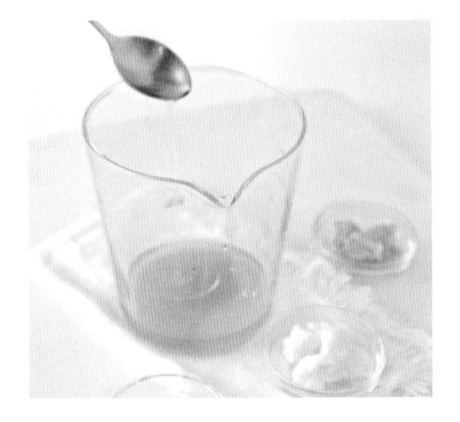

Step 2

Measure the rose water into a heatproof jug, add the contents of the astragalus capsule; stir. Add the Phase 3 ingredients; place the jug in a pan of simmering water.

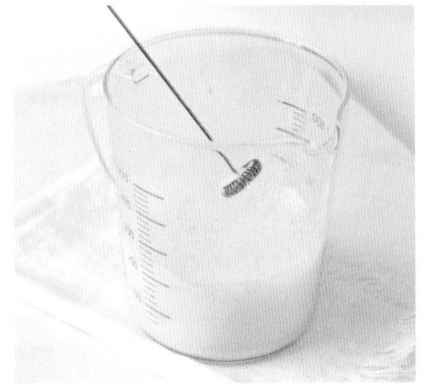

Step 3

Heat the jug with contents to 70–80°C (158–176°F). After 30 minutes, remove from the heat. Whizz with a milk frother. De-aerate and cool to 40°C (104°F).

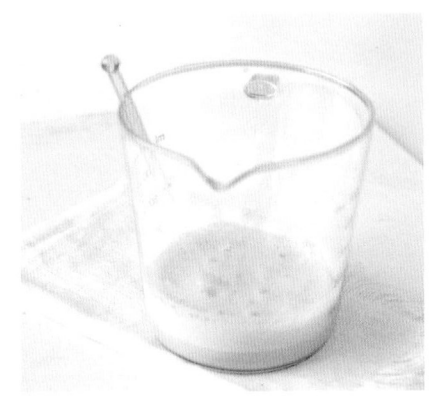

Step 4

Add the evening primrose mix and rosehip oil, then finally the geranium oil and preservative. Stir to mix and pour into a sterilized, airtight jar. Label as usual.

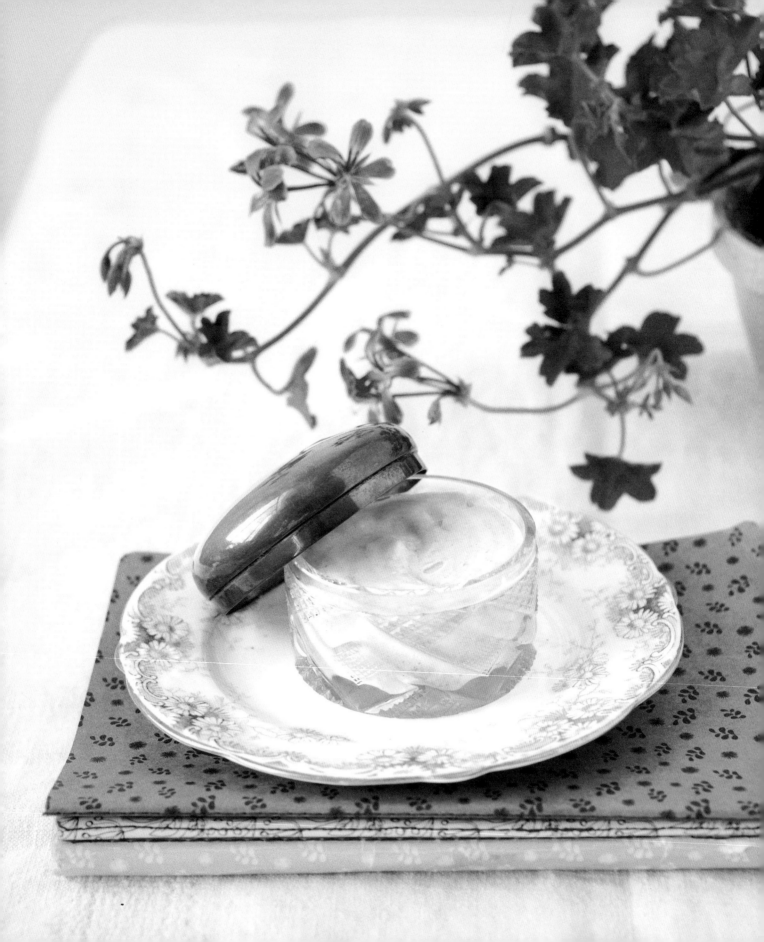

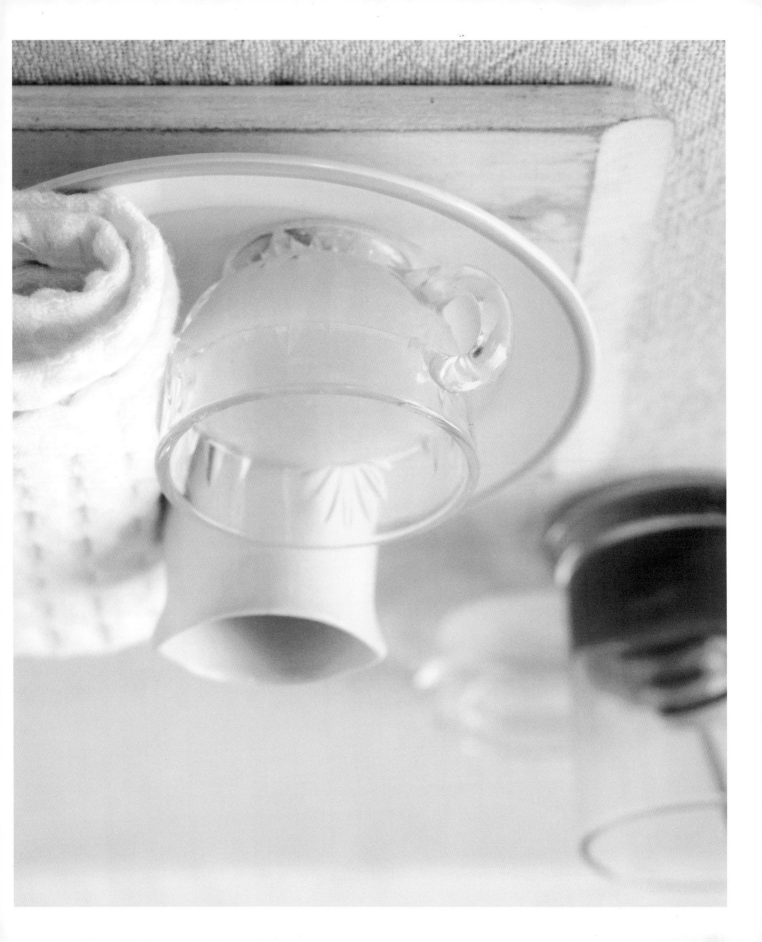

Gentle Dispersing Face Scrub/Mask with Vitamin C, Manuka Honey and Papaya

Face scrubs don't need to be harshly abrasive; this one has a mild exfoliating action. It contains manuka honey, which has moisturizing properties, and vitamin C powder and papaya enzyme, which brighten the skin by gently exfoliating dead cells. The addition of the honey to a Sucragel base brings a light beige colour to the product, but it will darken naturally over time.

Makes approx. 50g (1¾oz)

INGREDIENTS
Phase 1
2g (½ tsp) manuka honey
45ml (3 tbsp) Sucragel CF base

Phase 2
2 papaya enzyme tablets
 (2 x 60mg)
1g (¼ tsp) vitamin C powder
2 drops sweet orange essential oil

SPECIAL EQUIPMENT
small heatproof dish
small pestle and mortar

SAFE STORAGE
Store in a cool, dry place away from sunlight. Keeps for up to 3 months.

HOW TO APPLY
Apply a small amount to damp skin, avoiding the eyes, then massage gently. Rinse with warm water.

Tip!
This product can also be used as a leave-on mask. Apply a thin layer to clean skin, avoiding the eyes, and leave for 5 minutes. Remove with a warm, damp facecloth.

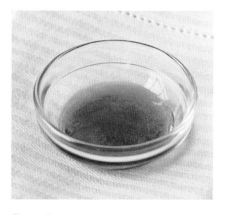

Step 1
Melt the honey very gently in a small heatproof dish; don't cook! Use a warming drawer if your cooker has one; otherwise, a few minutes in a cool oven will work.

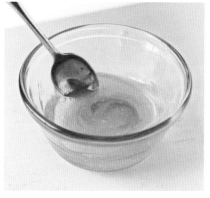

Step 2
Measure the Sucragel CF base into a small bowl (see page 43 for the method). Gradually mix the honey into the gel, stirring slowly.

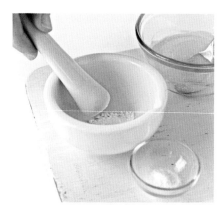

Step 3
Using a pestle and mortar, crush the papaya enzyme tablets into a fine powder, then add the vitamin C powder. Add the powder mix to the gel in the bowl.

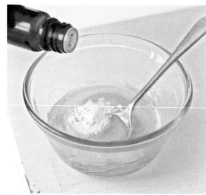

Step 4
Add the sweet orange oil and stir, ensuring you remove any lumps from the powder. Spoon into a sterilized, airtight jar. Label with the date and ingredients used.

Face Mask with Clay and Camomile Tea

(for dry or mature skin)

Use this soothing clay-based mask to perk up dry or mature skin. ESP Organic SafeEmuls SCA and Emulsifying Wax BP are excellent emulsifiers for making oil-into-water creams and lotions without the need for specialized mixers. SafeEmuls, however, has a more natural but odoriferous content.

Makes approx. 70g (2½oz)

INGREDIENTS
10g (¼oz) kaolin (white clay)
   or green clay
35ml (2¼ tbsp) camomile tea;
   40ml (2¾ tbsp) if using
   Emulsifying Wax BP
10g (¼oz) ESP Organic SafeEmuls
   SCA or 5g (1 tsp) Emulsifying
   Wax BP
10ml (2 tsp) olive oil
4ml (¾ tsp) glycerine
5 drops camomile essential oil
   in dilution
10 drops grapefruit seed extract
   (as a preservative)

SPECIAL EQUIPMENT
small heatproof dish
small teapot
strainer
thermometer

SAFE STORAGE
Store in a cool, dry place away from sunlight. Keeps for up to 3 months.

HOW TO APPLY
Apply to clean skin, avoiding the eyes, and leave for 5–10 minutes. Rinse with water.

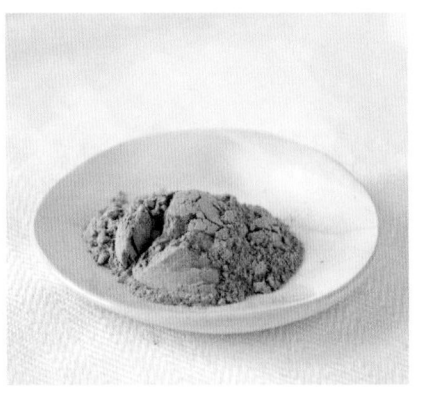

Step 1
Put the clay in a small heatproof dish and place for 30 minutes in an oven heated to 100–120°C (212–248°F) to ensure that the powder is sterile.

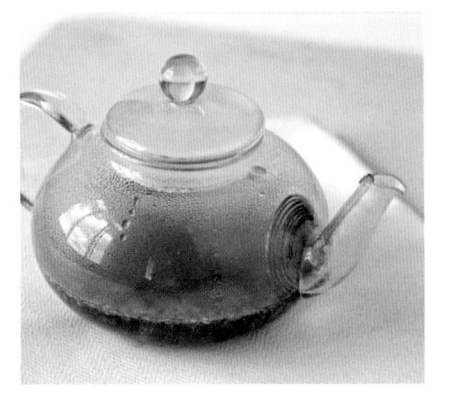

Step 2
Make the camomile tea as per the instructions on the packet, and infuse for at least 10 minutes in a teapot. Strain once infused and set the liquid aside.

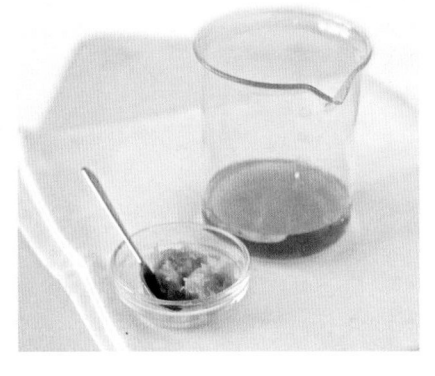

Step 3
Weigh the ESP Organic SafeEmuls SCA (or Emulsifying Wax BP), olive oil and glycerine into a heatproof jug; mix with the camomile tea. Place in a pan of simmering water and heat to 70–80°C (158–176°F).

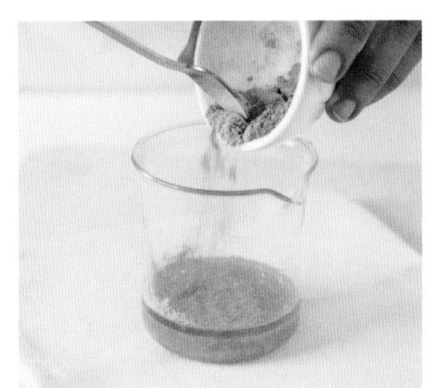

Step 4
Remove from the heat after 30 minutes and cool to around 40–50°C (104–122°F), then add the clay, camomile oil and preservative. Mix until smooth, then pour into a sterilized, airtight jar. Label as usual.

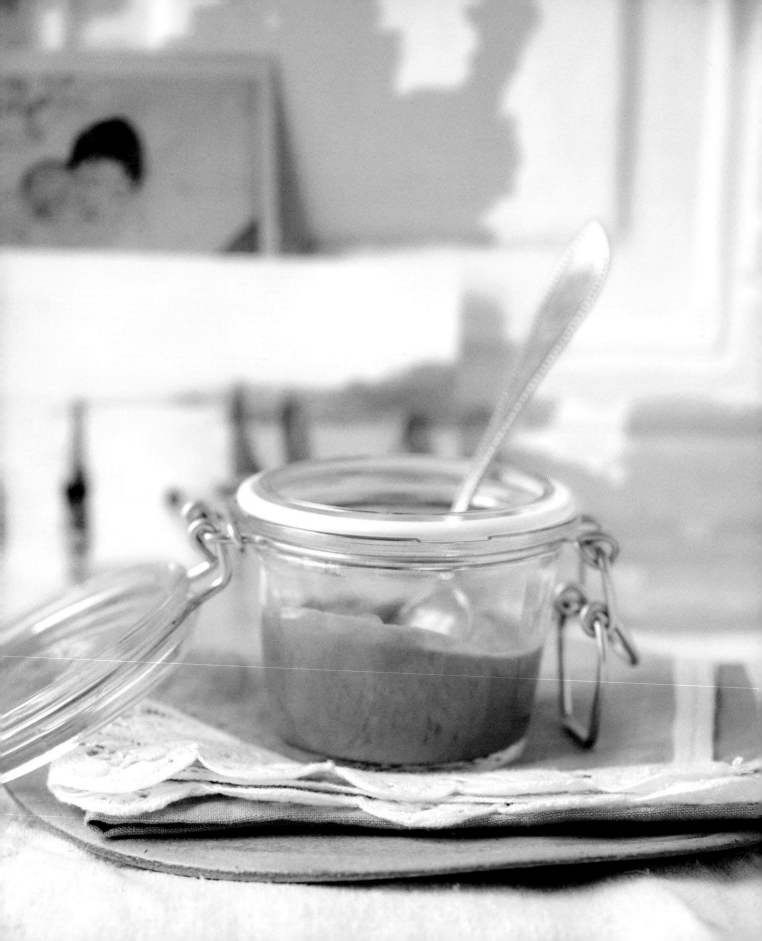

Fresh and Instant Pineapple and Yoghurt Smoothie Clay Mask

Feel free to raid the fridge – to make a simple, fresh face mask. The thick consistency of Greek yoghurt, which helps both to tighten pores and smooth fine lines, is particularly suited to a mask. Pineapple is excellent as a skin-brightening and exfoliating ingredient owing to the bromelain enzyme found in the fruit. However, it is very powerful and not recommended for sensitive skin.

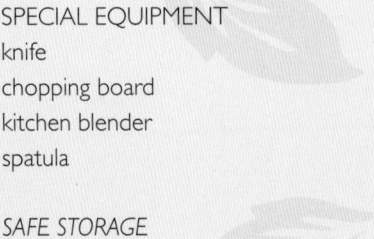

Makes approx. 100g (3½oz)

INGREDIENTS
5 × 2.5-cm (1-inch) fresh pineapple
   chunks
2 tbsp Greek yoghurt
2 tbsp aloe vera juice
kaolin (white clay), to required
   consistency*

* Try substituting kaolin with coconut flour or, for drier skin, oat flour.

SPECIAL EQUIPMENT
knife
chopping board
kitchen blender
spatula

SAFE STORAGE
Make and use fresh. Keeps for up to 3 days when stored in the fridge.

HOW TO APPLY
It will smell deliciously of pineapple, but don't be tempted to drink the mask! Use immediately. Apply to clean skin, avoiding the eyes, and leave for only a few minutes, removing the mixture as soon as the skin feels tight or sensitized; 3–5 minutes will be enough for most normal to oily skins. Rinse off with plenty of warm water and pat skin dry. Any remaining mixture can be stored in the fridge, but should be used within a few days.

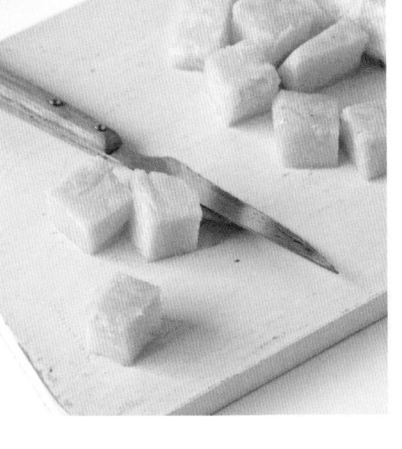

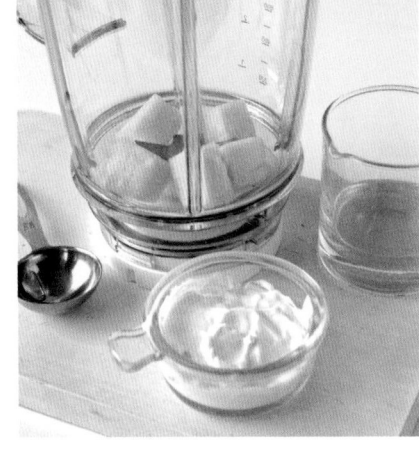

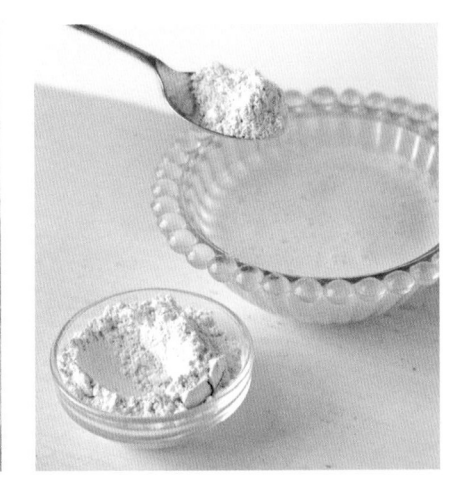

Step 1
Peel and chop the pineapple into 2.5-cm (1-inch) chunks. Don't worry too much about the precise size of the chunks, but make sure you chop off any tough core.

Step 2
Place the pineapple, Greek yoghurt and aloe vera juice in a blender and blitz until smooth. Using a spatula, transfer the mixture into a small bowl.

Step 3
Add the kaolin to make a smooth, semi-thick consistency, stirring with a stainless steel teaspoon. The mask will be a soft yellow colour and resemble a smoothie.

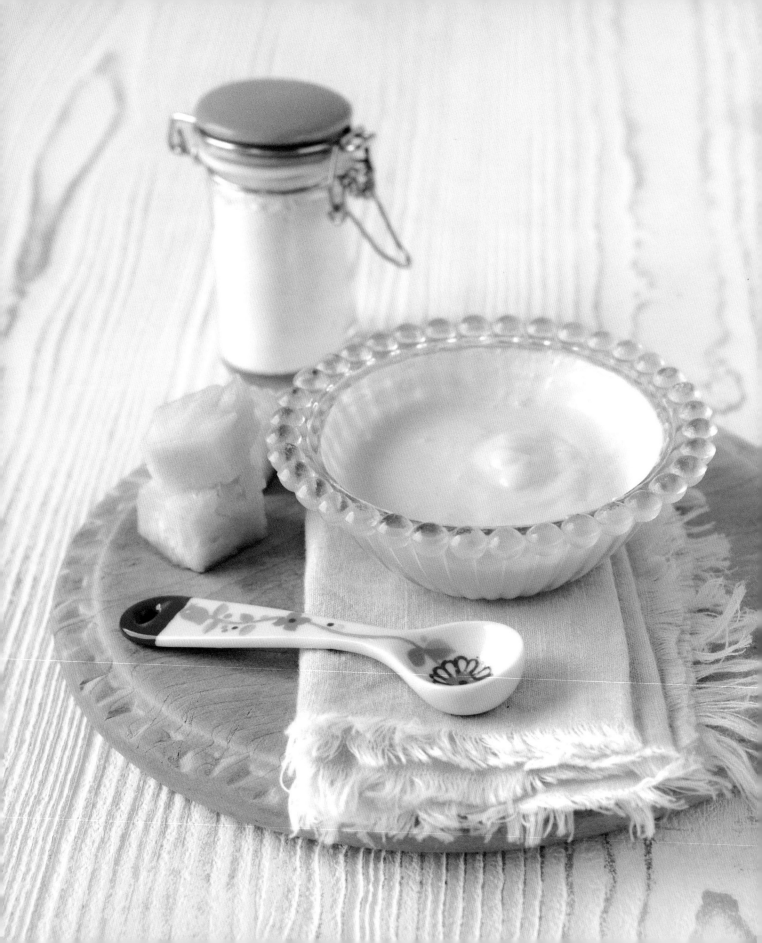

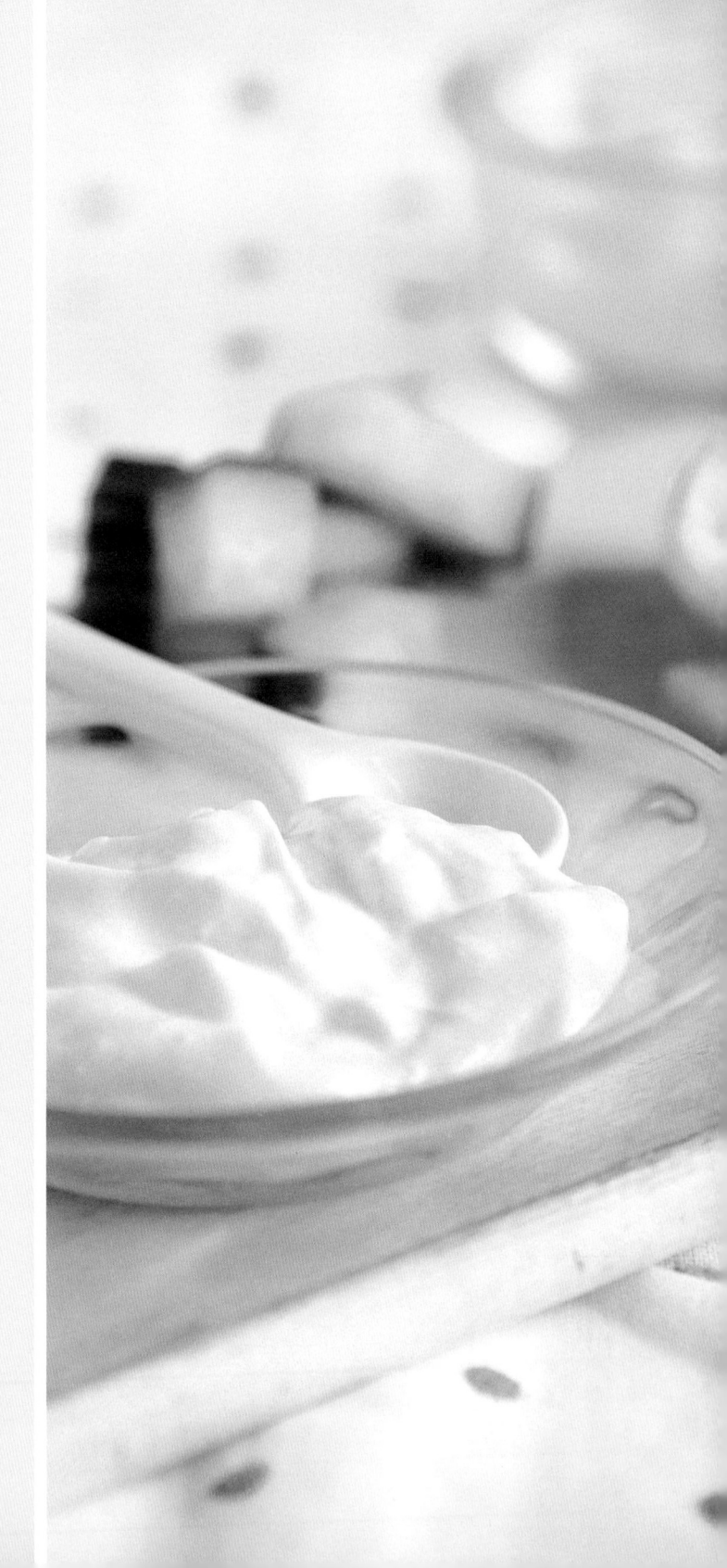

Adaptation:

Instant Anti-Pigmentation Mask with Yoghurt, Cucumber and Elderflower

Cucumber, lemon and elderflower have been used for centuries as naturally brightening ingredients in skincare. This recipe can be made without elderflowers, if unavailable.

Makes approx. 100g (3½oz)

INGREDIENTS
5 x 2.5-cm (1-inch) cucumber chunks
optional: 1 fresh head of elderflowers
   or 1 tbsp dried elderflower
2 tbsp Greek yoghurt
2 tbsp aloe vera juice
2 drops lemon essential oil

Chop the cucumber chunks and (if using) elderflowers very finely. Mix with the Greek yoghurt, aloe vera juice and lemon oil in a small bowl, mashing the cucumber with a fork to release its juice. If you are using dried elderflower, leave the mixture for 10–15 minutes to allow the elderflower to soften slightly in the yoghurt. If you wish, you can put the mixture in a blender and whizz for a few seconds to obtain a smoother consistency.

SAFE STORAGE
Make and use fresh. Keeps for up to 3 days when stored in the fridge.

HOW TO APPLY
Use immediately. Apply to clean skin, avoiding the eyes, and leave for around 10 minutes, until the mask begins to tighten. Rinse off with plenty of warm water and pat skin dry. Any remaining mixture can be stored in the fridge, but should be used within a few days.

Cooling Gelatine Mask with Chlorella and Gotu Kola

This gel mask uses leaf gelatine. Normally associated with making desserts, gelatine lends itself well to this kind of application, and you can add different ingredients to the basic method (see Step 8). Because the recipe is left to set in the fridge in the final stage, it becomes a cool, invigorating mask that also has a tightening effect on the skin. Gotu kola has anti-inflammatory and anti-ageing properties, and chlorella, which is derived from algae, can help to reduce skin redness.

Makes approx. 250g (8¾oz)

INGREDIENTS
1 gotu kola tablet (250mg)
1 chlorella tablet (500mg)
250ml (8½fl oz) aloe vera juice
1–2 leaves gelatine (generally to be used in 250ml (8½fl oz) liquid, but check manufacturer's instructions)
10 drops camomile essential oil in dilution

SPECIAL EQUIPMENT
small pestle and mortar
dish of water (in which to soak gelatine)
optional: stick blender or milk frother

SAFE STORAGE
Make and use fresh. Keeps for up to 3 days when stored in the fridge.

HOW TO APPLY
Use immediately. Apply to clean skin, avoiding the eyes, and leave for around 10 minutes or until the mask feels set. A cooling and tightening effect will be particularly noticeable with the gel version. Rinse off with plenty of warm water and pat skin dry. Any remaining mixture can be stored in the fridge, but should be used within a few days.

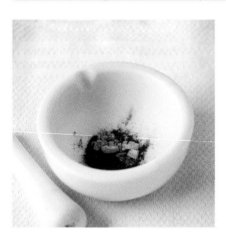

Step 1
Crush the gotu kola and chlorella tablets using a pestle and mortar. Try to eliminate as many lumps as possible, to make a fine powder.

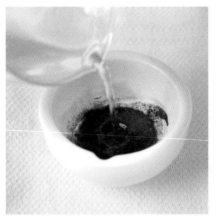

Step 2
Measure the aloe vera juice into a jug, then pour a small amount into the mortar and mix into the powder with a stainless steel teaspoon to make a thick paste.

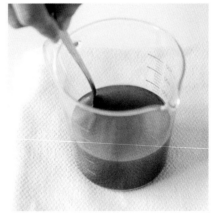

Step 3
Add the aloe vera, gotu kola and chlorella mixture from the mortar to the jug containing the remaining aloe juice, and stir to mix.

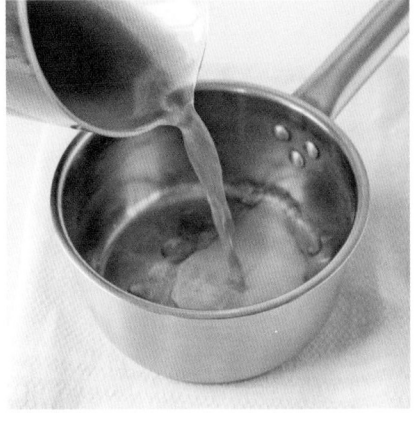

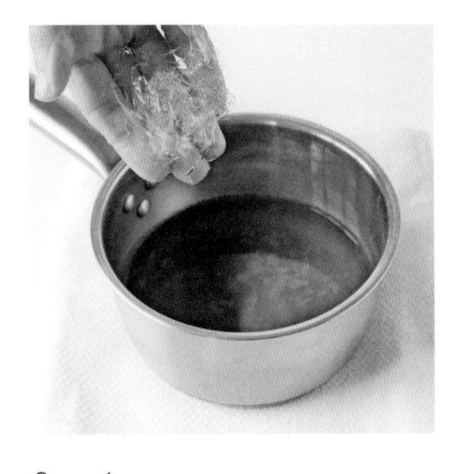

Step 4
Place the gelatine leaf in a dish (1 leaf for a soft gel; 2 for a thicker consistency), and add enough water to cover completely. Allow to soak for 5 minutes or until supple (following the manufacturer's instructions).

Step 5
Pour the aloe vera, gotu kola and chlorella mixture into a stainless steel pan and heat – but be careful not to boil – the liquid. Remove the pan from the heat.

Step 6
Remove the gelatine from the water, squeeze to remove liquid, then add to the heated liquid in the pan. Stir briefly to mix, then pour the liquid from the pan into a bowl or jar.

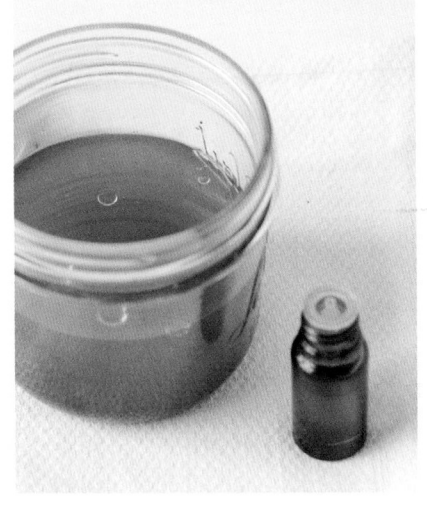

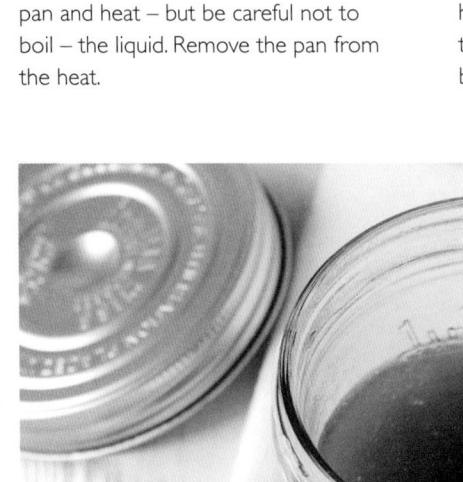

Step 7
Allow to cool, then add the camomile oil. Stir and place in the fridge for about an hour to set.

Step 8
Remove the gel from the fridge once it is set, and stir to ensure it is well mixed, and the gotu kola and chlorella are not sitting at the bottom. You can keep the mask as a clear green gel or add a face lotion or cream to make it a moisturizing 'mousse' mask. A recipe such as Fresh and Light

Shea Butter Face Cream (page 66) or Face Lotion with Thyme and Grapefruit (page 70) would be ideal. Simply add approximately 3 teaspoons of face cream/lotion to 50ml (3½ tbsp) of gel in the jar and whizz with a stick blender or milk frother to mix thoroughly.

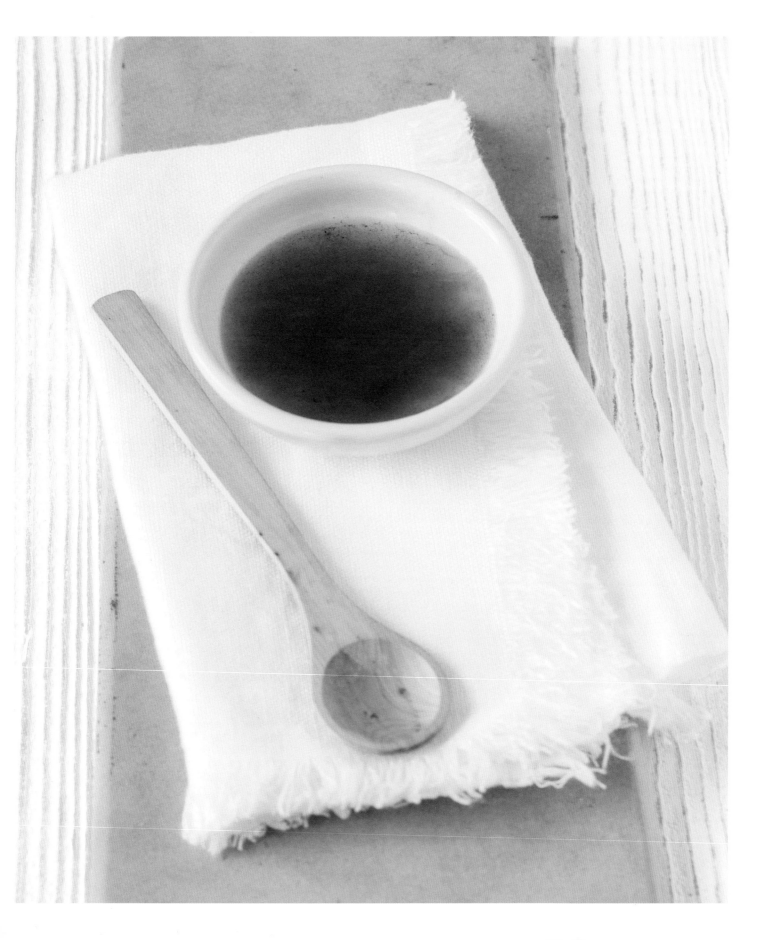

Eye Cream with Rosehip, Evening Primrose and Rhodiola

Our quickly absorbed eye cream is packed with high-performing natural ingredients, including rhodiola, which has been found to protect skin from environmental damage and to reduce the appearance of fine lines. Note that the recipe makes enough cream for two small jars or bottles.

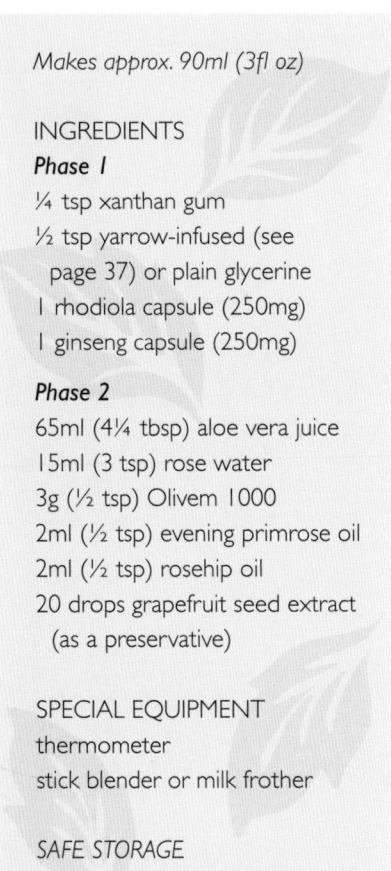

Makes approx. 90ml (3fl oz)

INGREDIENTS
Phase 1
¼ tsp xanthan gum
½ tsp yarrow-infused (see
    page 37) or plain glycerine
1 rhodiola capsule (250mg)
1 ginseng capsule (250mg)

Phase 2
65ml (4¼ tbsp) aloe vera juice
15ml (3 tsp) rose water
3g (½ tsp) Olivem 1000
2ml (½ tsp) evening primrose oil
2ml (½ tsp) rosehip oil
20 drops grapefruit seed extract
    (as a preservative)

SPECIAL EQUIPMENT
thermometer
stick blender or milk frother

SAFE STORAGE
Store in a cool, dry place away from
sunlight. Keeps for up to 3 months.

HOW TO APPLY
Using your ring finger, gently pat a small
amount on to moisturized skin around
each eye, either in the morning or at night.

Step 1

Combine the Phase 1 ingredients in a small beaker or measuring glass and mix until smooth. Try to eliminate lumps from the xanthan gum and to disperse evenly the contents of the two capsules.

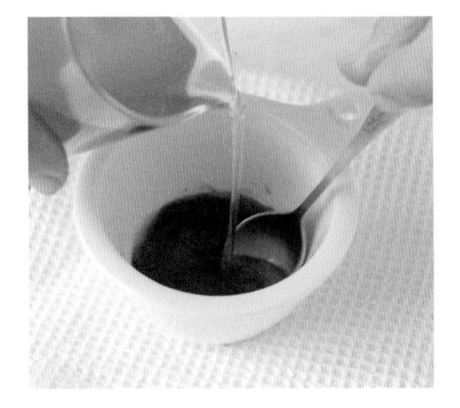

Step 2

Measure the aloe vera juice and rose water into a heatproof jug. Slowly add this liquid to the beaker to dilute the Phase 1 ingredients. Mix well, then return the whole liquid to the heatproof jug.

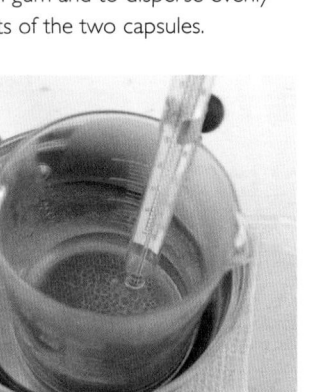
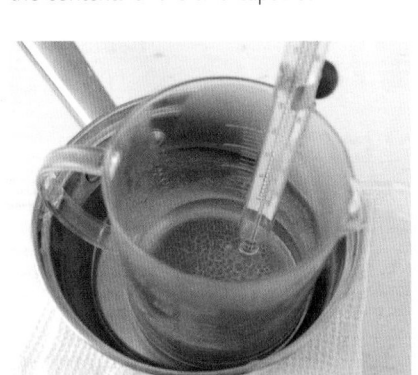

Step 3

Add the Olivem 1000 and both Phase 2 oils. Place the jug in a pan of simmering water; heat to 70–80°C (158–176°F) for 30 minutes, then remove from the heat.

Step 4

Whizz with a milk frother and allow to de-aerate then cool to around 50°C (122°F). Add the preservative, then pour into a sterilized, airtight jar. Label as usual.

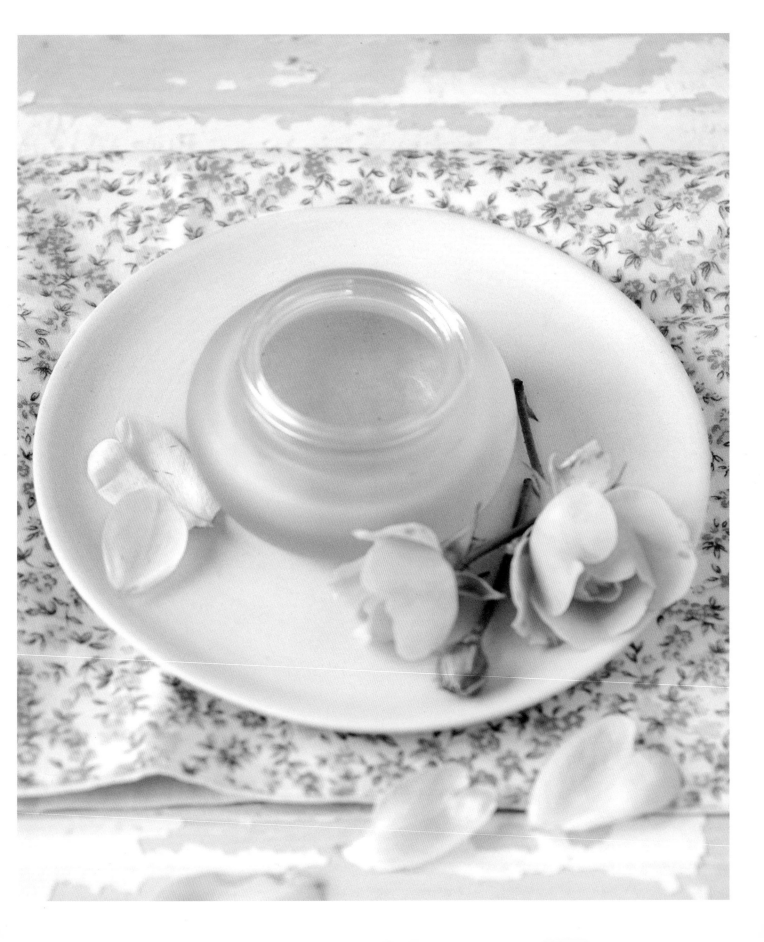

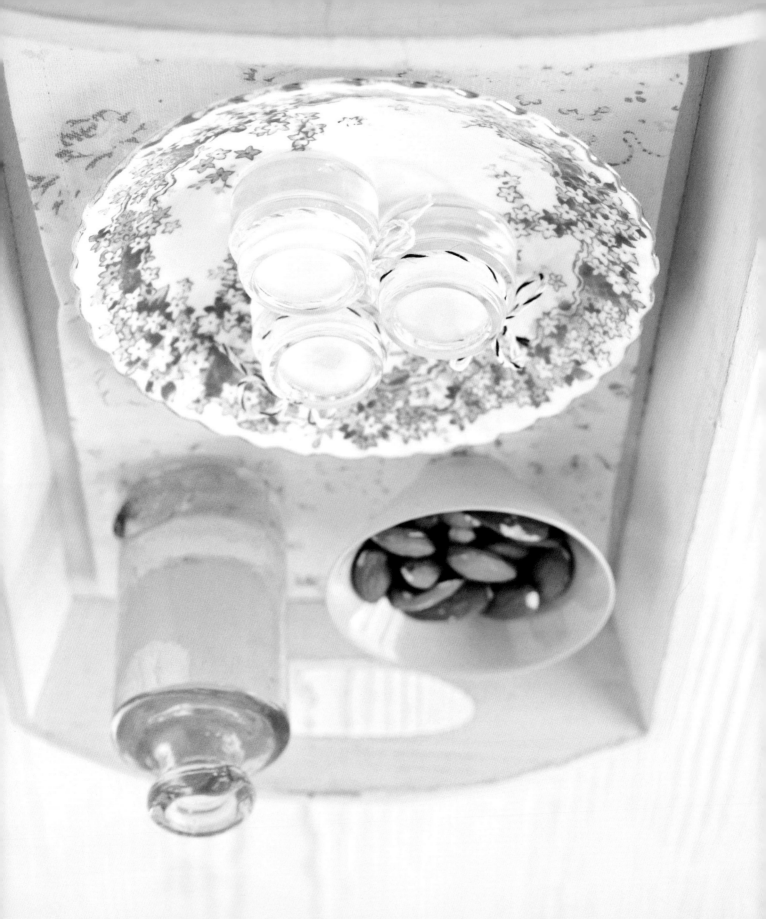

Trio of Lip Balms

Lip balms are indispensable, so it's great to have a quick and easy recipe to make your own favourite or try out a new flavour. We have suggested three versions: sweet (but not overpowering) Banoffee, irresistible Coconut and Almond, and fresh Cool Lips Spearmint and Shea Butter. The natural base of sweet almond oil and beeswax creates a moisturizing balm to soothe the lips. This recipe makes at least a couple of small pots, so you could make one for a friend or just store a spare in a handy place.

INGREDIENTS

Banoffee
Makes approx. 18g (½oz)
8ml (1½ tsp) wheatgerm oil
8ml (1½ tsp) sweet almond oil
2g (½ tsp) beeswax white BP
2 drops banana food flavour*
2 drops caramel food flavour*

Coconut and Almond
Makes approx. 17g (½oz)
8g (1½ tsp) unrefined coconut oil
8ml (1½ tsp) sweet almond oil
1g (¼ tsp) beeswax white BP
10 drops almond extract
  flavouring*

Cool Lips Spearmint and Shea Butter
Makes approx. 17g (½oz)
10ml (2 tsp) sweet almond oil
1g (¼ tsp) beeswax white BP
6g (1¼ tsp) shea butter
4 drops spearmint essential oil

SPECIAL EQUIPMENT
No special equipment required.

* Food flavours can vary in strength, so these amounts are a guide. Experiment with a couple of drops initially and increase if necessary.

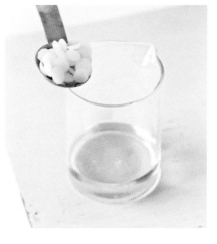

Step 1
Weigh all the ingredients except the flavours/spearmint oil into a heatproof jug. Place the jug in a pan of simmering water and heat until the beeswax is molten.

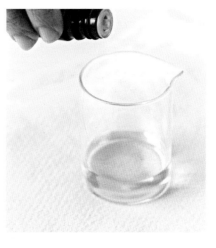

Step 2
When the ingredients are fully melted, remove the jug from the pan, allow the mixture to cool slightly and then add the flavours or spearmint oil. Stir to mix well.

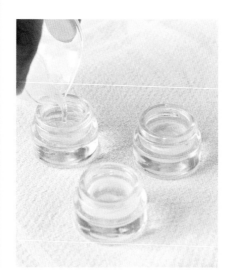

Step 3
While the mixture is still hot and liquid, pour into small sterilized, airtight pots or jars to set. Once cool, label with the date and ingredients used.

HOW TO APPLY
Dab a small amount on to the lips as often as required.

SAFE STORAGE
Store in a cool, dry place away from sunlight. Keeps for up to 6 months.

Lip and Cheek Tint

This balm with a hint of colour is a variation on the straightforward lip balm (page 89) and is almost as easy to make. Four to five drops of natural food colouring are sufficient to gain a touch of colour on the lips and cheeks. Adding more colour will result in a deeper shade, but the effect on the skin will be a lot more translucent and subtle than it appears in the container. Note, however, that it may be a process of trial and error finding a food colour that dissolves successfully in oil. At our local supermarket we found two colourants that resulted in fabulous shades of pink and coral. This is a particularly great project to try with teenagers in order to get them started with handmade cosmetics.

Makes approx. 18g (½oz)

INGREDIENTS
15ml (3 tsp) sweet almond oil
1g (¼ tsp) shea butter
2g (½ tsp) beeswax white BP
4–5 drops (as preferred) natural
   food colouring

SPECIAL EQUIPMENT
optional: glass rod

SAFE STORAGE
Store in a cool, dry place away from sunlight. Keeps for up to 6 months.

HOW TO APPLY
Apply to the lips as often as required. Or, using your fingertips, pat a small amount in circular motions on to the apples of your cheeks (the fleshy parts most prominent when you smile). Gradually add more tint until you have a lovely rosy glow. Remember that it's easier to add more product than it is to remove it!

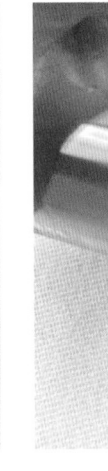

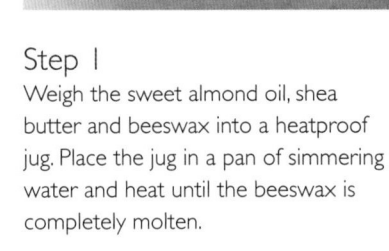

Step 1
Weigh the sweet almond oil, shea butter and beeswax into a heatproof jug. Place the jug in a pan of simmering water and heat until the beeswax is completely molten.

Step 2
When the ingredients are fully melted, remove the jug from the pan, allow the mixture to cool slightly and then add the food colouring a drop at a time to obtain the desired depth of colour. Stir to mix.

Step 3
While the mixture is still hot and liquid, pour into small sterilized, airtight pots or tins to set. You should get a smooth, even finish on the surface. Once cool, label with the date and ingredients used.

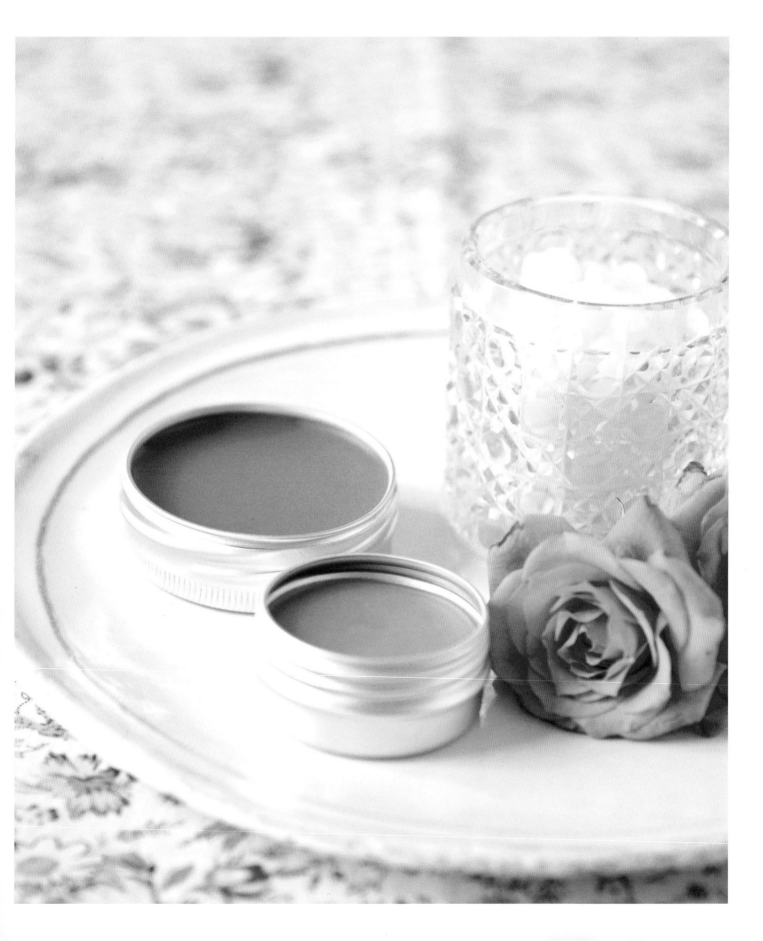

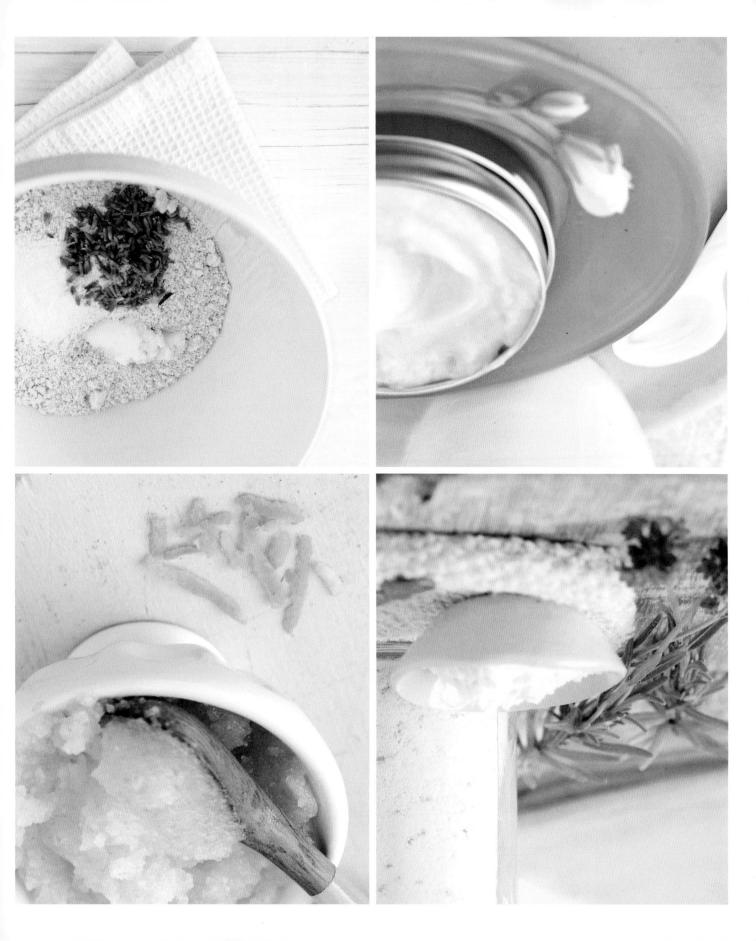

BODY

Lavender and Rosemary Bath Soak with Milk Powder

The rich blend of milk powder and sweet almond oil in this recipe helps to soften and condition the skin. Epsom salts are detoxifying, and the essential oil of lavender will soothe the senses after a long day. Rosemary leaves are optional and add a lovely, fresh herbal scent to the powder.

Makes approx. 200g (7oz)

INGREDIENTS
178g (6¼oz) dried milk powder
4g (¾ tsp) unperfumed soap
10g (¼oz) Epsom salts
4ml (¾ tsp) sweet almond oil
optional: 1 tsp dried rosemary
  leaves
20 drops lavender essential oil
20 drops rosemary essential oil
40 drops grapefruit seed extract
  (as a preservative)

SPECIAL EQUIPMENT
baking tray (cookie sheet)
chopping board
grater
mixing bowl or Kilner jar, for mixing

SAFE STORAGE
Store in a cool, dry place away from sunlight. Keeps for up to 3 months. If you are using fresh rosemary, store in the fridge for up to 3 days.

HOW TO USE
Add a few spoonfuls to warm running water, then relax in the bath for at least 20 minutes.

Tip!
If available, fresh rosemary is a great substitute for dried leaves; it will make the powder really fragrant and refreshing. The leaves should be washed and dried before use. Fresh leaves are heavier than dried, so you can add slightly more in weight. Chop very finely with a kitchen knife or scissors.

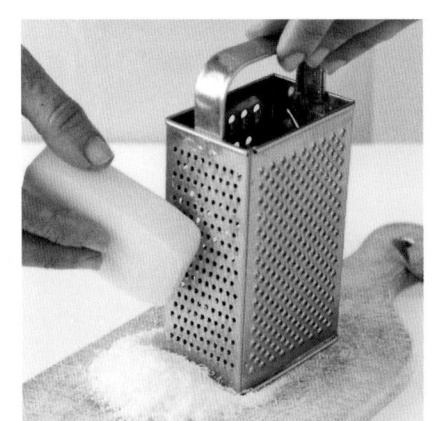

Step 1
Pour the milk powder on to a baking tray (cookie sheet) and place in an oven heated to 100°C (212°F) for 30 minutes to destroy any microbes. Remove and set aside to cool.

Step 2
Over a chopping board, grate the soap using the fine side of a grater. Set aside. Weigh the remaining ingredients, including the dried or fresh rosemary leaves (if using), into a bowl or a sterilized Kilner jar.

Step 3
Add the cooled milk powder and grated soap to the bowl or jar, and stir to mix thoroughly. Pour into a sterilized, airtight jar, or seal in the Kilner jar. Label with the date and ingredients used.

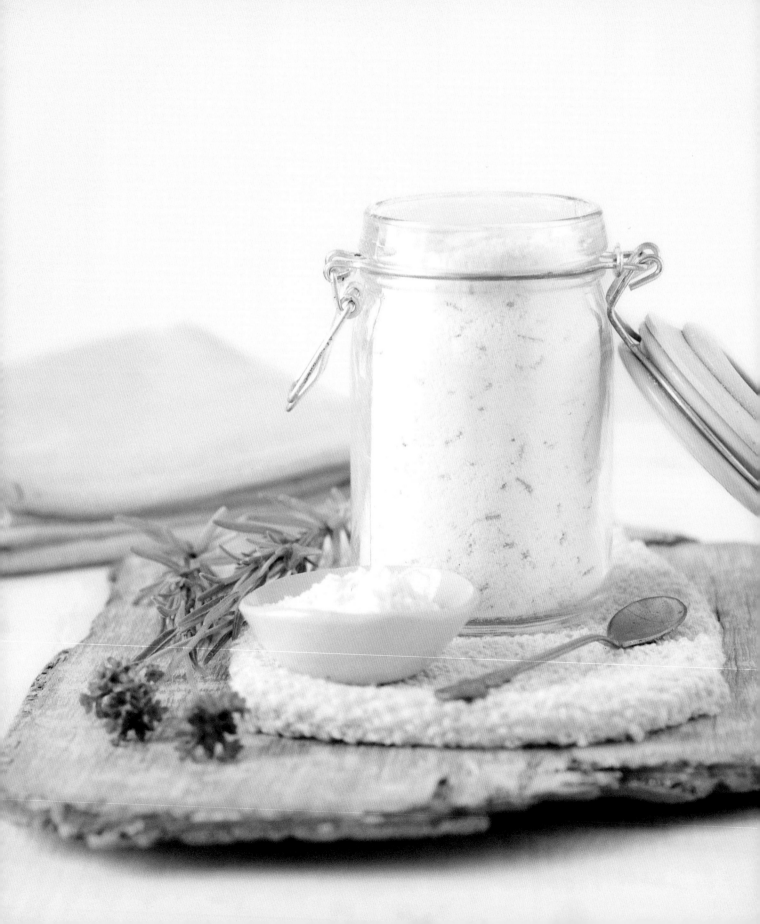

Bath Bombs with Flower Petals

Makes approx. 455g (16oz)

INGREDIENTS
1–2 handfuls dried petals
250g (8¾oz) sodium
  bicarbonate (baking soda)
125g (4½oz) citric acid
50g (1¾oz) cornflour
  (cornstarch)
5ml (1 tsp) fragrance or
  essential oils (see Step 3)
25ml (5 tsp) distilled witch
  hazel BPC

SPECIAL EQUIPMENT
optional: small pestle and mortar
large mixing bowl
vinyl gloves (see Step 2)
optional: plastic pipette
plant-mister/other spray bottle
moulds
palette knife
chopping board

SAFE STORAGE
Store in a cool, dry place away
from sunlight. Keeps for up to
12 months.

HOW TO USE
Leave for 24 hours in a warm, dry place
before wrapping in circles of cellophane
tied with pretty ribbon (see page 138).

Depending on the size of the mould, drop
one or two bombs into warm running
water. The bombs will fizz as they hit
the water, leaving it softened, fragranced
and with a fine sprinkling of floating petals.

Bath bombs may sound daunting to make, but in fact this is a very simple recipe using kitchen-cupboard basics, jazzed up with the addition of flowers from the garden (see Step 1 for suggested dried petals to use). Because it's such a hands-on project, it's a great way to get children and teenagers started with making cosmetics at home. Bath bombs make a wonderful, inexpensive gift; you can really use your imagination to make them special.

Depending on the size of the moulds you use, the recipe will make quite a large number of bombs. If you can find some vintage tart tins or chocolate moulds, you can create bombs with delightful embossed patterns. Failing that, use any small bun tins or even individual silicone muffin moulds.

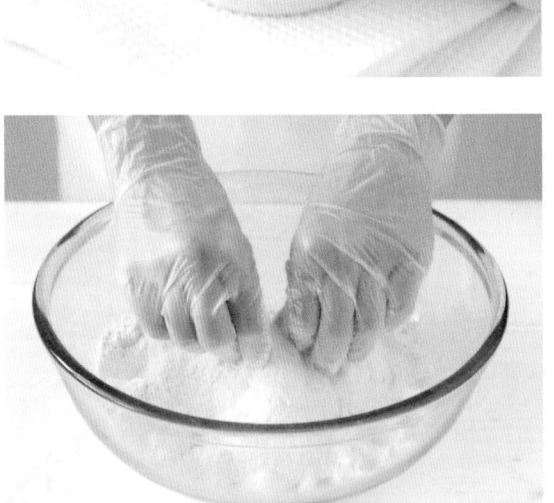

Step 1
Tear the dried petals to ensure they are small in size; about 1cm (just under ½ inch) long is best. Alternatively, crush them using a pestle and mortar. Suitable dried petals include red rose (not pink, as they will discolour), lavender and calendula (marigold). See the instructions on page 20 for drying petals.

Step 2
Place the dry ingredients (but not the petals) in a large mixing bowl and, wearing disposable vinyl gloves, mix together with your hands and fingers to ensure there are no lumps. The gloves will help to protect your hands from the powders, which can become slightly abrasive, particularly during prolonged mixing.

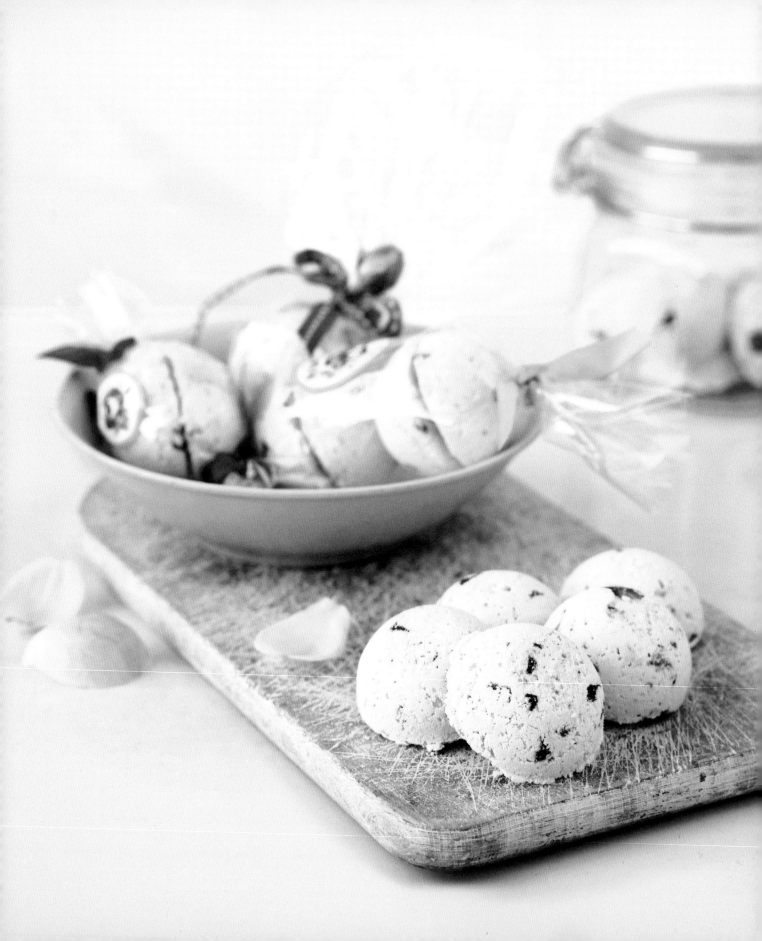

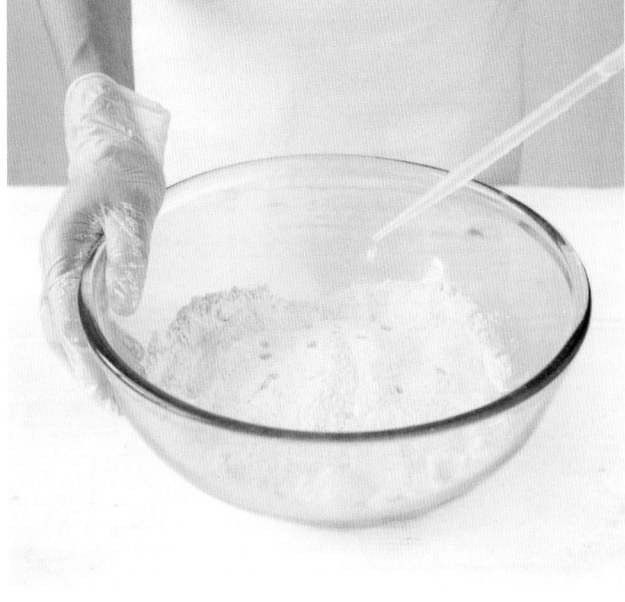

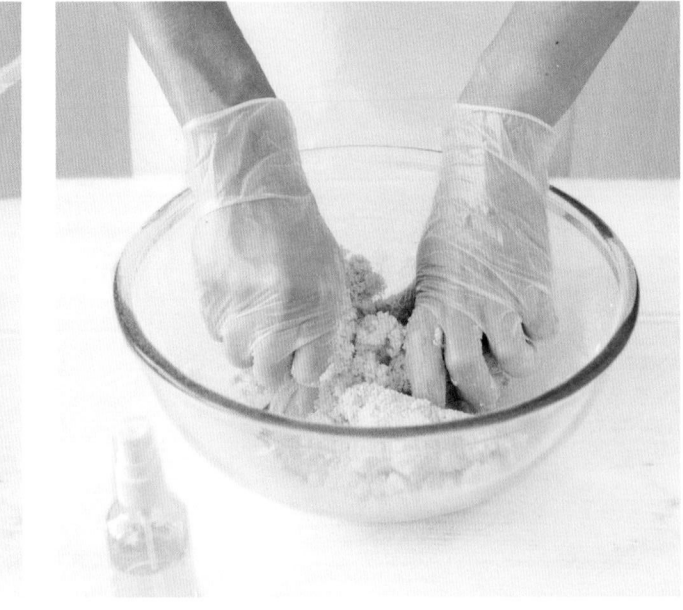

Step 3

Add the essential oils or, using a plastic pipette, the fragrance, and mix with your hands to ensure even distribution in the mixture. If you are using fragrance, ensure it is suitable for cosmetic use.

Step 4

Spray the witch hazel into the mix a little at a time, until the mixture resembles damp sand and forms clumps when squeezed in the hands.

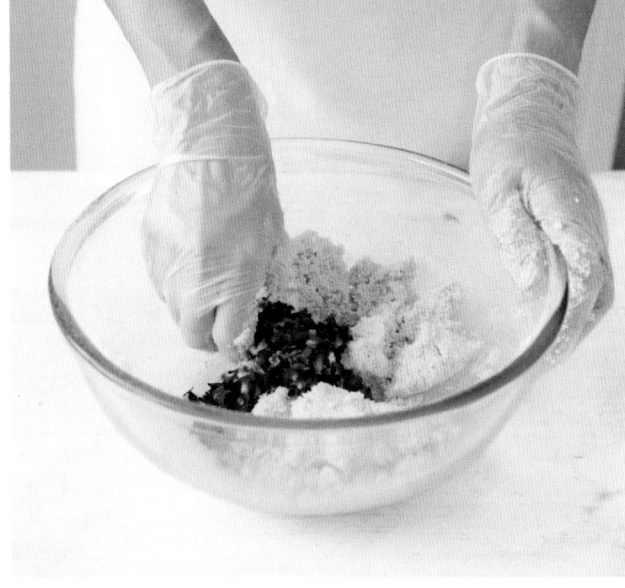

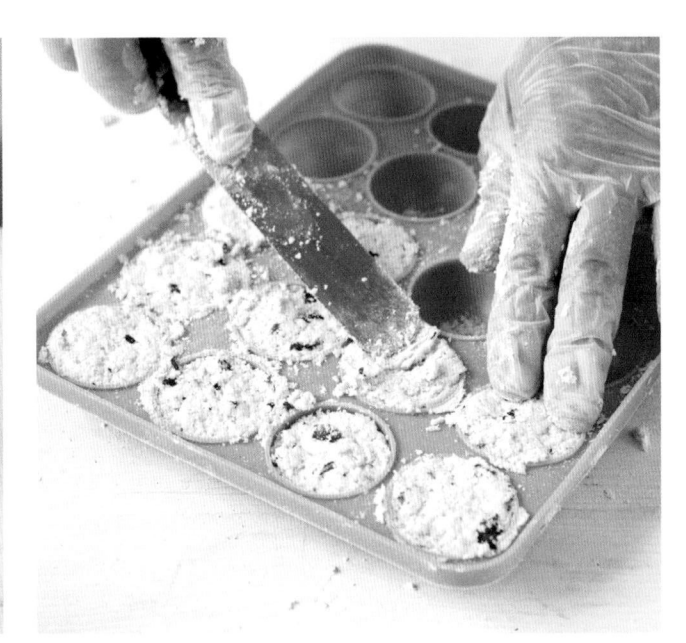

Step 5

Mix in the petals. The amount is down to personal preference (1–2 handfuls should be sufficient), but the aim is to have some petals in each bath bomb.

Step 6

Press the mixture into the moulds until each bomb is level with the top of the mould. Make sure the mixture is really compacted. Smooth the surface with a palette knife to ensure it is flat.

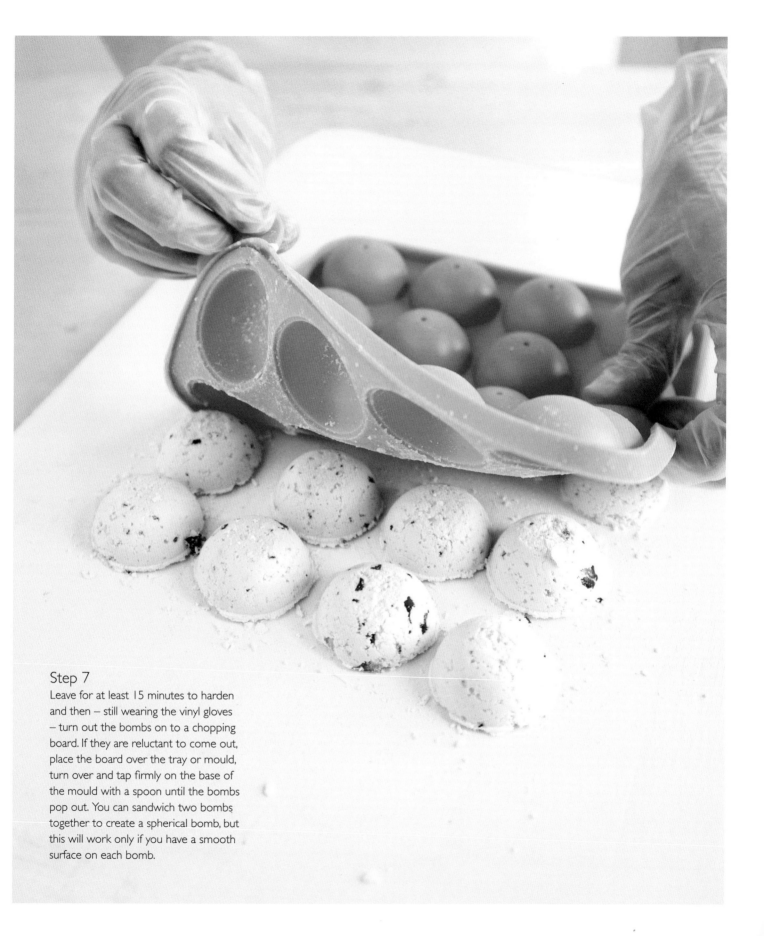

Step 7

Leave for at least 15 minutes to harden and then — still wearing the vinyl gloves — turn out the bombs on to a chopping board. If they are reluctant to come out, place the board over the tray or mould, turn over and tap firmly on the base of the mould with a spoon until the bombs pop out. You can sandwich two bombs together to create a spherical bomb, but this will work only if you have a smooth surface on each bomb.

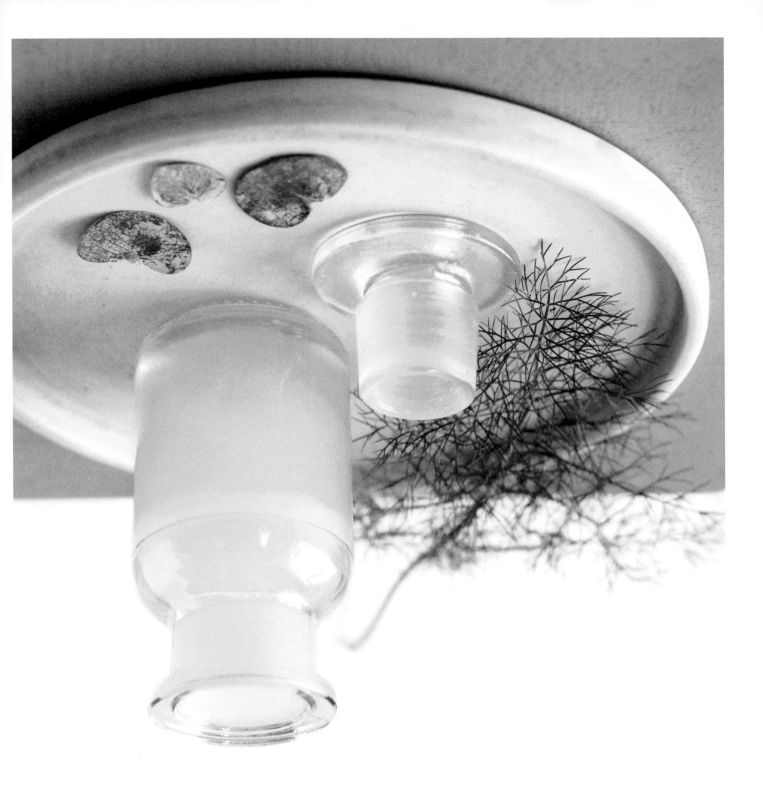

Seaweed and Herb Bath Essence

Seaweed is a wonderful natural ingredient for skincare products. It contains vitamins, minerals and antioxidant compounds that have been found to be beneficial in hydrating and repairing the skin. For this bath essence we use serrated wrack, but you can use other varieties. Harvest the seaweed from the shore or, ideally for freshness, close to the tidal edge. You'll need a couple of handfuls for this recipe.

Makes approx. 200ml (7fl oz)

INGREDIENTS
98ml (6½ tbsp) seaweed infusion
  (see Steps 1 and 2)
80ml (5½ tbsp) Plantapon LGC
10ml (2 tsp) Lamesoft PO 65
10ml (2 tsp) infused or plain
  glycerine (see Step 3)
10 drops eucalyptus essential oil
10 drops fennel essential oil
10 drops juniper essential oil
10 drops thyme essential oil
40 drops grapefruit seed extract
  (as a preservative)

SPECIAL EQUIPMENT
scissors
chopping board
thermometer
colander (strainer) or sieve
  (sifter)

SAFE STORAGE
Store in a cool, dry place away from sunlight. Keeps for up to 3 months.

HOW TO USE
Pour 1–2 capfuls (approx. 5–10ml) into warm running water, then relax in the softly foaming and clean-scented bathwater for an indulgent 20 minutes or so.

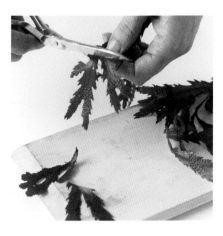

Step 1
Wash a couple of handfuls of seaweed thoroughly and cut into lengths of about 5–7cm (2–3 inches). Place the seaweed in a stainless steel pan and cover with water.

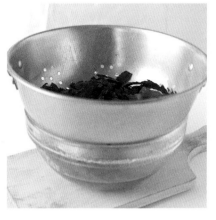

Step 2
Bring to the boil and cook at 70–80°C (158–176°F) for 30 minutes. Remove from the heat and allow to cool. Drain the seaweed pieces and retain the infusion.

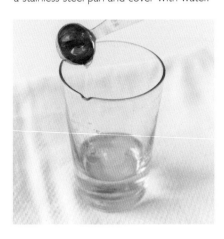

Step 3
Mix the Plantapon LGC and Lamesoft PO 65 together in a beaker or jug. Add the plain glycerine or, if you prefer, a rosemary or thyme infusion (see page 37).

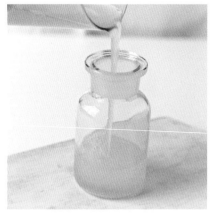

Step 4
Add 98ml (6½ tbsp) of the seaweed infusion, then the essential oils and preservative. Stir to mix, then pour into a sterilized bottle and seal. Label as usual.

Dispersing Bath Oil with Citrus and Juniper

This dispersing oil will delicately scent the bathwater with the aroma of citrus and juniper, to refresh and revive the weary. This is an especially easy recipe to make because it requires no heating; it stores well and, presented in a pretty glass bottle, would make an elegant gift. Unlike in non-dispersing bath oils, the polysorbate enables the rice bran oil and essential oils to disperse evenly throughout the water and on to your skin, leaving it feeling silky and perfectly moisturized. Another undisputed benefit is that you don't have to scrub to remove any oily residue left around the bathtub. Who wants to spend time doing that chore after a relaxing soak!

Makes approx. 100ml (3½fl oz)

INGREDIENTS
85ml (5¾ tbsp) rice bran oil
10ml (2 tsp) polysorbate 20
40 drops tangerine essential
  oil
40 drops lemon essential oil
20 drops juniper essential oil

SPECIAL EQUIPMENT
optional: plastic pipette
optional: funnel

SAFE STORAGE
Store in a cool, dry place away from sunlight. Keeps for up to 6 months.

HOW TO USE
Pour 2–3 capfuls (approx. 10–20ml) into warm running water. Set aside at least 20 minutes to relax in the bath and allow the uplifting scents of the essential oils to work their magic.

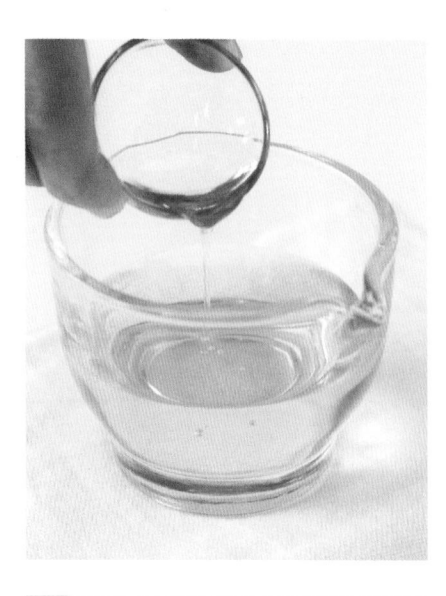

Step 1
First, check the odour of the rice bran oil to ensure the freshness. Avoid using oils with rancid odours, as this will spoil the fragrance of your finished product. Measure the rice bran oil and polysorbate 20 into a glass jug or beaker and stir together. The two liquids combine very easily to give a clear oil base.

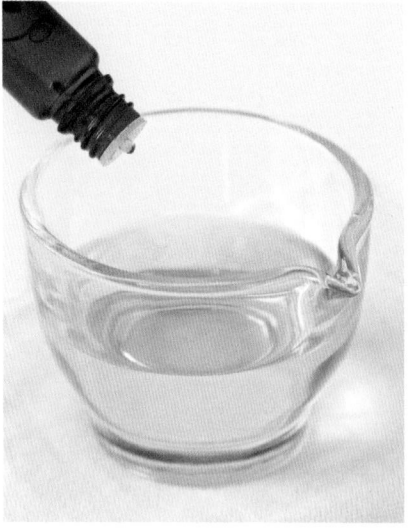

Step 2
Add the essential oils to the oil base using either a dropper bottle or a plastic pipette, and stir until the mix is completely clear. Pour into a sterilized, airtight glass bottle. You may find that the use of a small funnel helps the transfer. Label with the date and ingredients used.

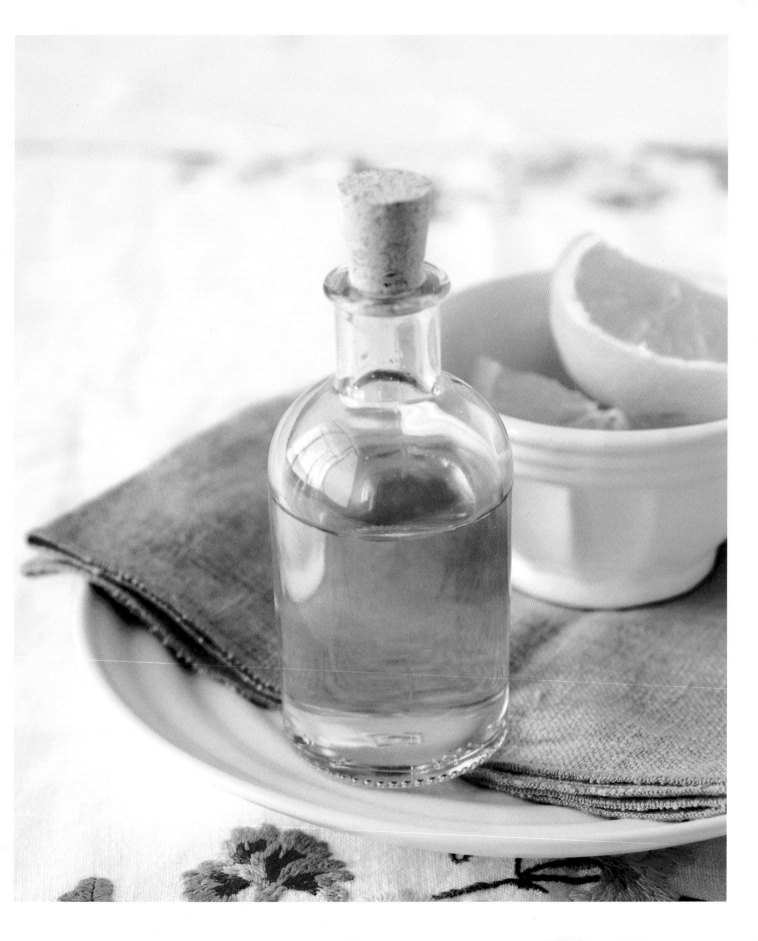

Sea Salt Body Scrub with Seaweed

Our marine-themed body scrub is not only exfoliating, on account of the mineral-rich salts and ground seaweed, but also moisturizing, owing to the high level of glycerine. If you don't have infused glycerine, simply substitute with plain. We've used bladderwrack, but you can use any seaweed, as long as it's thoroughly washed and dried before use. You'll need a couple of handfuls. The presence of the Olivem 1000 emulsifier allows the scrub to dissolve in water without leaving an oily film.

Makes approx. 200ml (7fl oz)

INGREDIENTS
10g (¼oz) ground bladderwrack
(or other seaweed; see Steps 1
and 2)
50g (1¾oz) sea salt crystals
10ml (2 tsp) rosemary-infused
glycerine (see page 37)
120ml (4fl oz) glycerine
8g (1½ tsp) Olivem 1000
20 drops lemon essential oil
10 drops pine essential oil

SPECIAL EQUIPMENT
colander (strainer)
baking tray (cookie sheet)
coffee grinder
thermometer
optional: stick blender or milk
frother

SAFE STORAGE
*Store in a cool, dry place away
from sunlight. Keeps for up to
6 months.*

HOW TO APPLY
*Massage into damp skin while in the bath
or shower, paying special attention to the
elbows, knees and feet. Rinse off thoroughly.
This also makes a great hand scrub.*

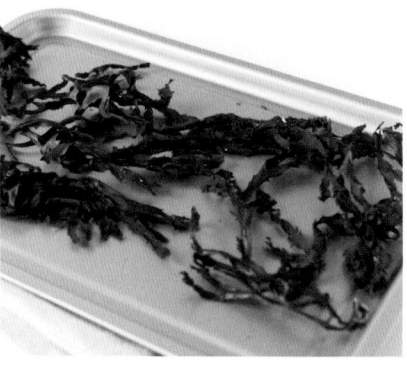

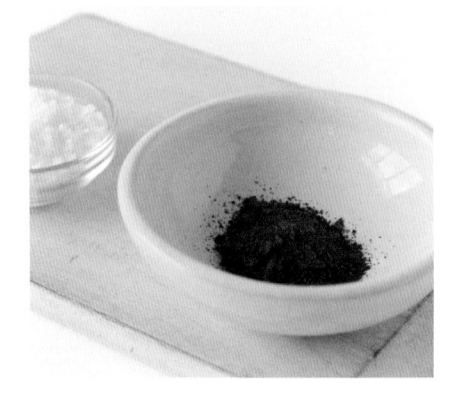

Step 1

Place a couple of handfuls of seaweed in a colander (strainer) and wash under plenty of clean, running water; then place on a baking tray (cookie sheet) in an oven heated to 120°C (248°F) for about 30 minutes until completely dry. Remove from the oven and set aside to cool.

Step 2

Blitz the cooled seaweed in a coffee grinder to make fine particles. Don't worry if it makes a loud noise in the grinder; bladderwrack is really hard when dry, which is why it makes a superb body exfoliant. If your sea salt is coarse, grind it as well, to make a smoother scrub.

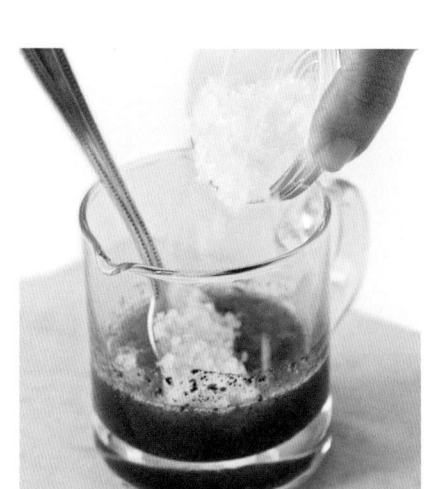

Step 3

Measure the glycerine (both infused and/or plain) into a heatproof jug and add the Olivem 1000. Place the jug in a pan of simmering water and heat to 75–80°C (167–176°F). Maintain this temperature for 30 minutes. Remove from the heat and allow to cool slightly. Stir vigorously to mix, or whizz briefly with a stick blender or milk frother. Add the salt and dried seaweed to the liquid and stir to mix. Finally, add the essential oils and then spoon into a sterilized, airtight jar. Label with the date and ingredients used.

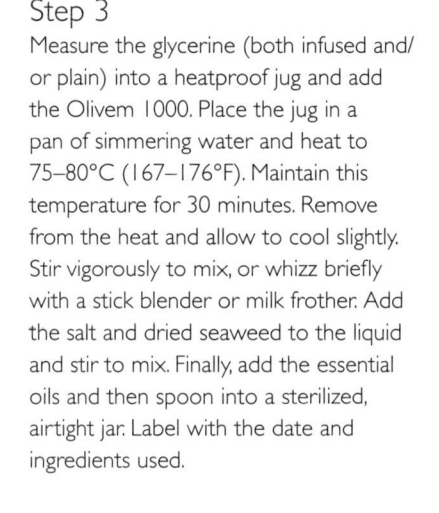

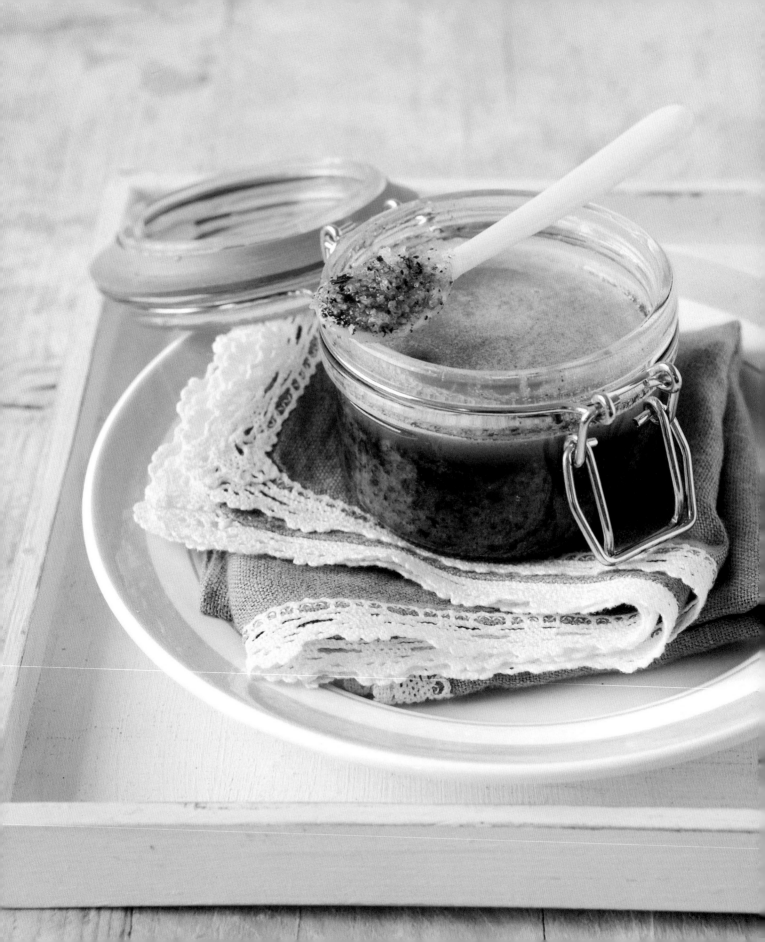

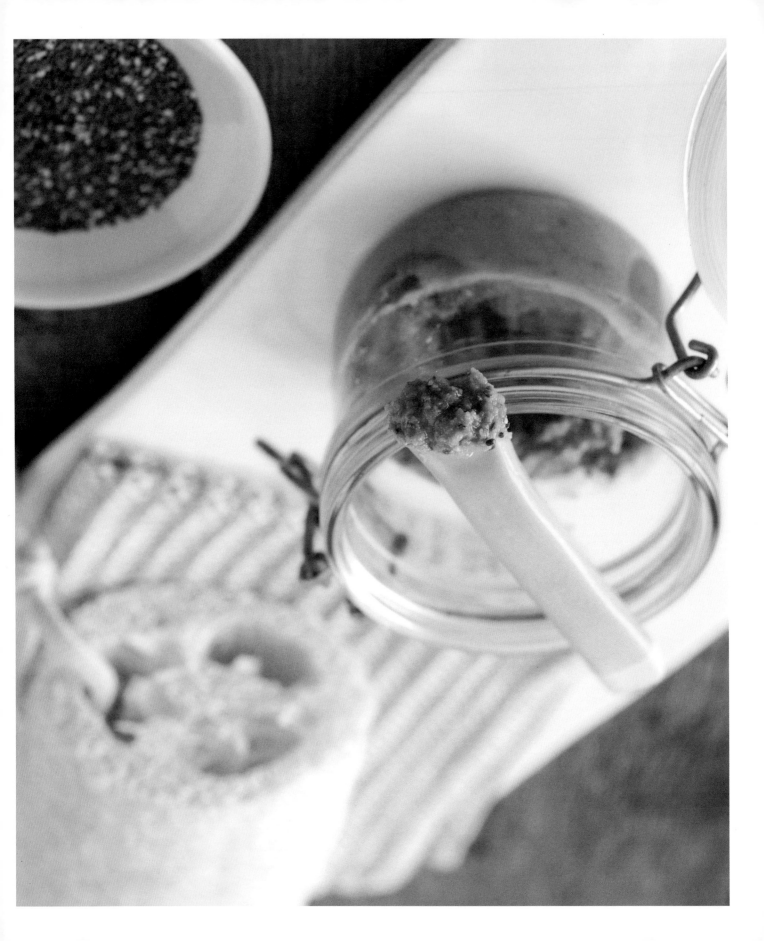

Dispersing Body Scrub with Chia Seeds and Pink Clay

A dusky shade of pink, this clay scrub is enriched with shea butter and natural oils to exfoliate and moisturize the skin. The petitgrain and lemongrass essential oils impart a zesty kick, making it perfect for use in your morning shower. The scrub is semi-solid, so is best scooped out of a jar or tub.

Makes approx. 200ml (7fl oz)

INGREDIENTS
16g (½oz) chia seeds
14g (½oz) pink clay
14g (½oz) shea butter
20g (¾oz) Olivem 1000
52ml (3½ tbsp) rice bran oil
28ml (5½ tsp) ivy-infused
   glycerine (see page 37)
10g (¼oz) unrefined coconut oil
24ml (4¾ tsp) jojoba oil
20g (¾oz) manuka honey
10 drops petitgrain essential oil
10 drops lemongrass essential oil

SPECIAL EQUIPMENT
small heatproof dish
thermometer
stick blender or milk frother

SAFE STORAGE
Store in a cool, dry place away from sunlight. Keeps for up to 1 month.

HOW TO APPLY
Massage into damp skin while in the bath or shower, paying special attention to the elbows, knees and other rough, dry patches. Rinse off; the scrub will leave a protective, moisturizing film on the skin. It is also suitable for use on very dry hands.

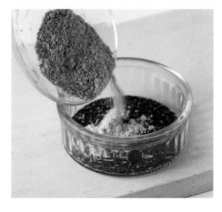

Step 1
Put the chia seeds and pink clay in a small heatproof dish and place in an oven heated to 100°C (212°F) for 30 minutes. Measure the remaining ingredients, apart from the essential oils, into a heatproof jug.

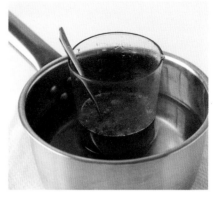

Step 2
Place the jug in a pan of simmering water and heat until the ingredients are molten (around 60–80°C/140–176°F), stirring well. Avoid overheating the honey so as to preserve its natural properties.

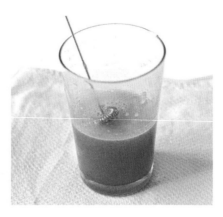

Step 3
Remove from the heat and whizz with a stick blender or milk frother. Cool slightly, then add the chia seeds and clay, then the essential oils, stirring to incorporate well.

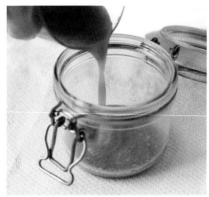

Step 4
Pour into a sterilized jar to set, but stir as the mixture begins to solidify to make sure that the seeds and clay are well distributed. Secure the lid, then label as usual.

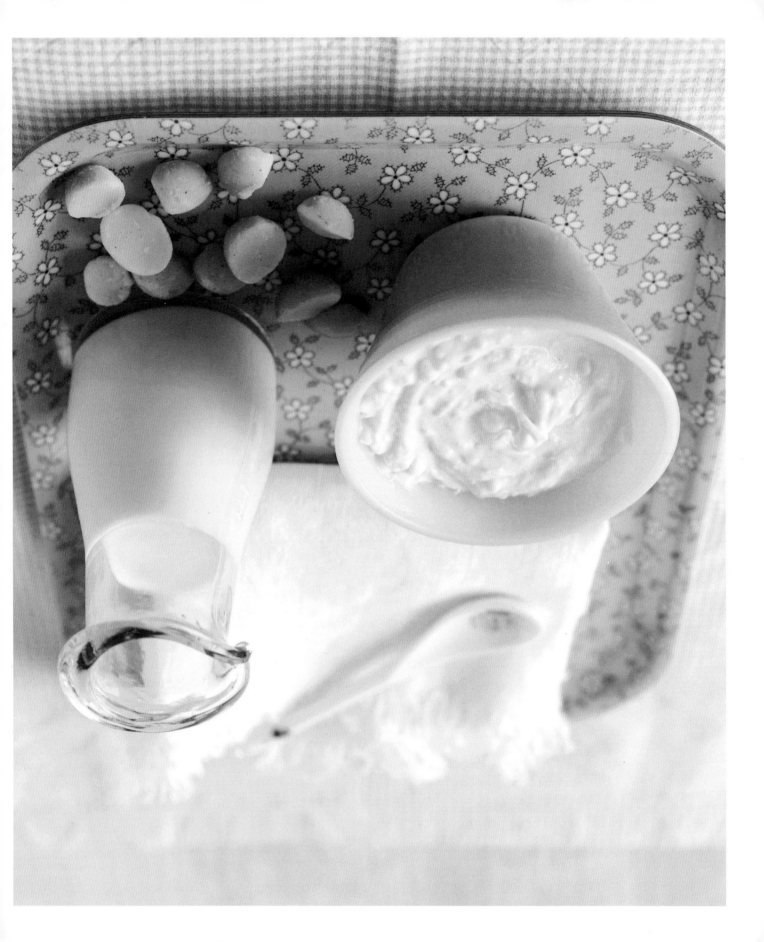

White Nut Body Butter

Makes approx. 200ml (7fl oz)

INGREDIENTS

Phase 1

20g (¾oz) ESP Organic SafeEmuls
  SCA

10g (¼oz) shea butter

10g (¼oz) cetearyl alcohol

4g (¾ tsp) beeswax white BP

24g (¾oz) unrefined coconut
  oil

24ml (4¾ tsp) macadamia
  nut oil

Phase 2

10ml (2 tsp) glycerine

1g (¼ tsp) xanthan gum

86ml (5¾ tbsp) rose water

10ml (2 tsp) coconut milk

20 drops ylang-ylang essential
  oil

60 drops grapefruit seed extract
  (as a preservative)

SPECIAL EQUIPMENT

thermometer

stick blender or milk frother

SAFE STORAGE

*Store in a cool, dry place away
from sunlight. Keeps for up to
3 months.*

HOW TO APPLY

*Apply a generous amount of butter to
slightly damp skin after a bath or shower,
and massage in gently. Leave to absorb for
a few minutes before getting dressed.*

This body butter contains a blend of luxurious, moisturizing white nut oils – coconut and macadamia – as well as coconut milk and shea butter. The addition of beeswax to the ESP Organic SafeEmuls SCA creates a rich consistency, which is a great treat for dry skin, while ylang-ylang essential oil lends an indulgent, tropical accent.

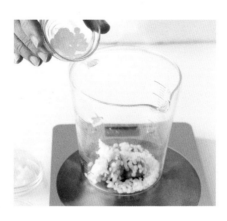

Step 1
Weigh the Phase 1 ingredients into a heatproof jug. Place the jug in a pan of simmering water and heat to 70–75°C (158–167°F), stirring until the wax melts.

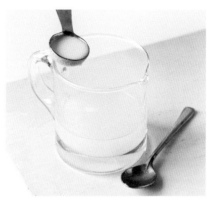

Step 2
Pour the glycerine and xanthan gum into a small measuring glass or beaker. Mix to form a paste, then incorporate the rose water and coconut milk. Mix until smooth.

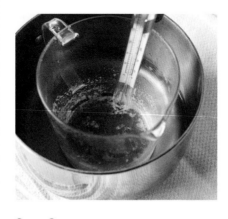

Step 3
Add the mixture in the glass to the jug. Stir and maintain the temperature at 70–75°C (158–167°F) for 30 minutes. Remove from the heat and whizz with a milk frother.

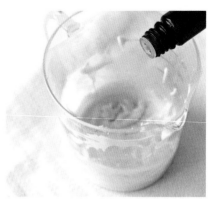

Step 4
Once the mixture has cooled to around 40°C (104°F), add the ylang-ylang oil and preservative, and stir to mix. Spoon into a sterilized, airtight jar. Label as usual.

Fresh Skin Body Lotion with Spearmint, Lime and Grapefruit

Our light and quickly absorbed lotion is easy to make, and the mint and citrus essential oils give it a lovely fresh, uplifting scent, especially in combination with the fragrant orange flower water. Ideal for use all over the body, it is particularly beneficial after your morning shower.

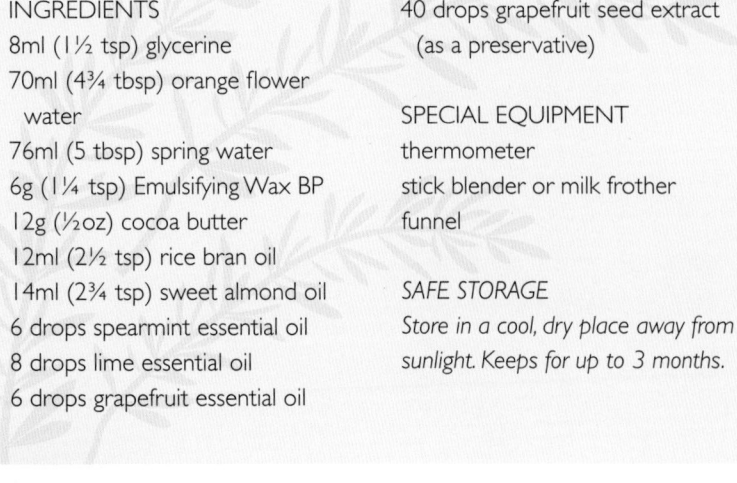

Makes approx. 200ml (7fl oz)

INGREDIENTS
8ml (1½ tsp) glycerine
70ml (4¾ tbsp) orange flower
    water
76ml (5 tbsp) spring water
6g (1¼ tsp) Emulsifying Wax BP
12g (½oz) cocoa butter
12ml (2½ tsp) rice bran oil
14ml (2¾ tsp) sweet almond oil
6 drops spearmint essential oil
8 drops lime essential oil
6 drops grapefruit essential oil

40 drops grapefruit seed extract
    (as a preservative)

SPECIAL EQUIPMENT
thermometer
stick blender or milk frother
funnel

SAFE STORAGE
Store in a cool, dry place away from sunlight. Keeps for up to 3 months.

HOW TO APPLY
Apply a generous amount of lotion to slightly damp skin after a bath or shower, and massage in gently. Leave to absorb for just a couple of minutes before getting dressed.

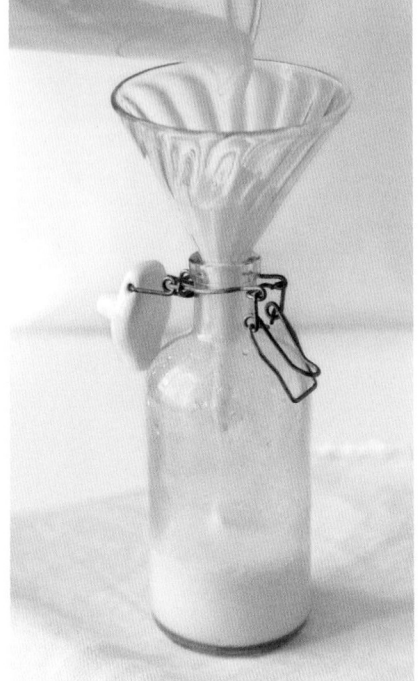

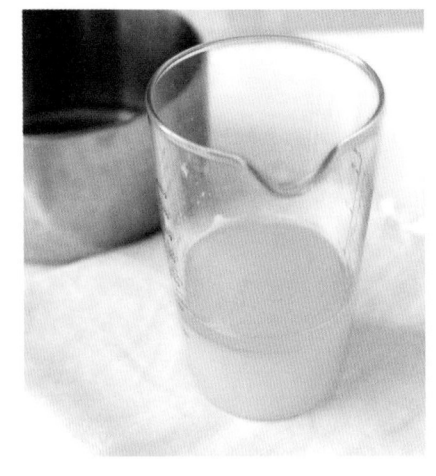

Step 1
Weigh all the ingredients except the essential oils and preservative into a heatproof jug. Heat in a pan of simmering water to 70–80°C (158–176°F).

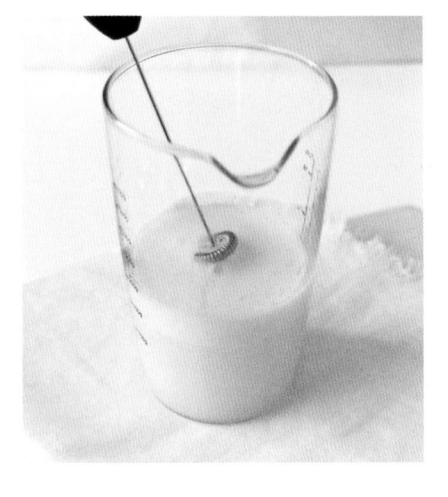

Step 2
Maintain the heat for 30 minutes, then remove the jug. The ingredients will have separated during heating (see Step 1 image). Whizz with a milk frother.

Step 3
Once the mixture has de-aerated and cooled to 40°C (104°F), add the essential oils and preservative. Stir, then funnel into a sterilized, airtight bottle. Label as usual.

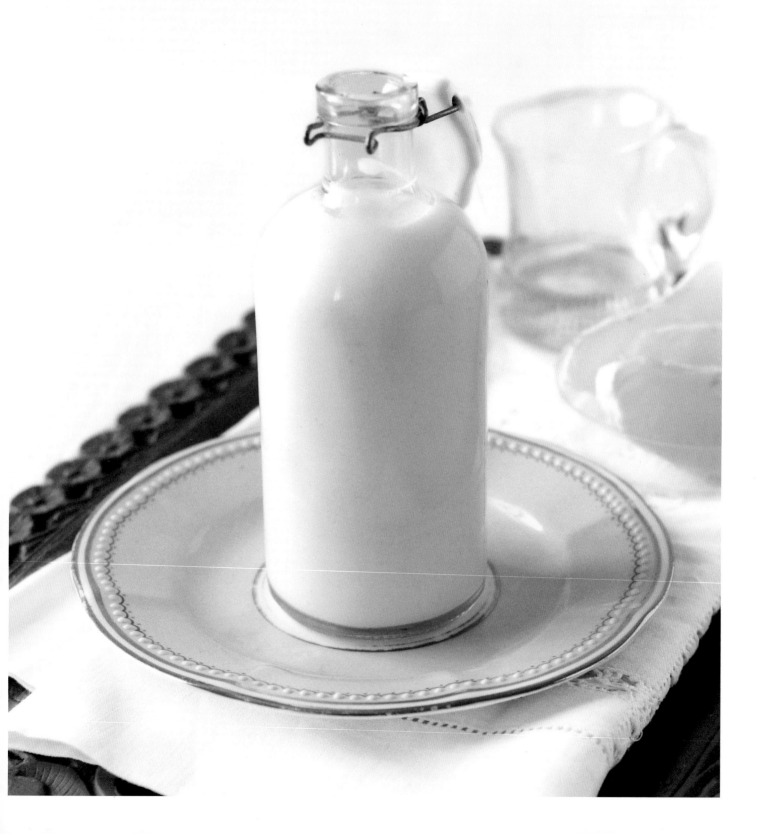

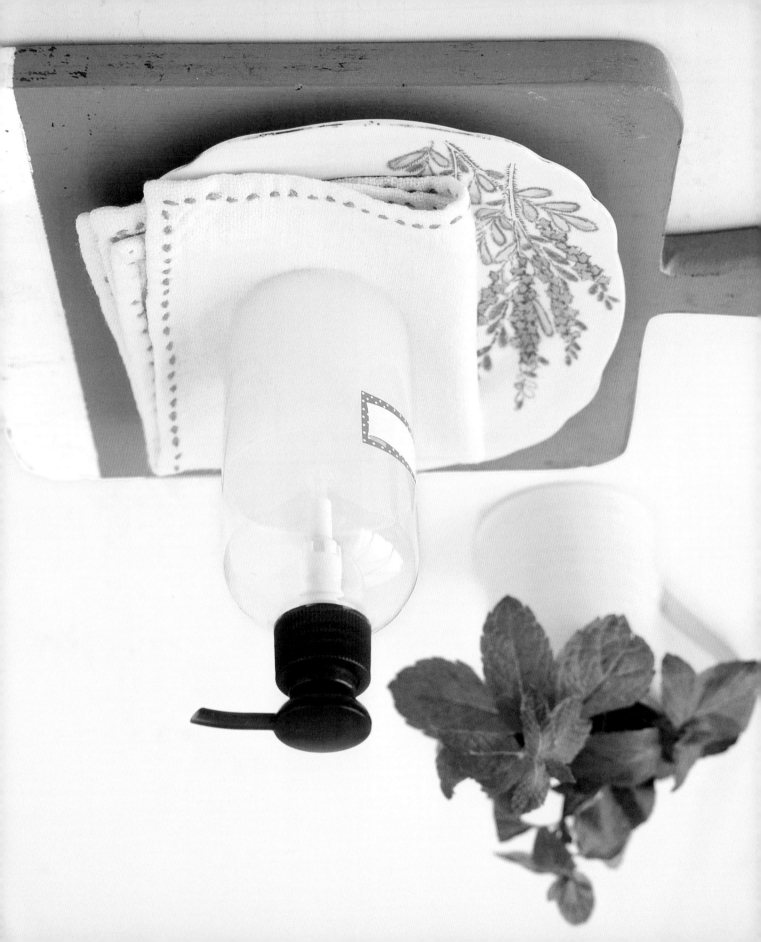

Hand and Body Wash with Rosemary, Mint and Basil

This refreshing hand and body wash is a great recipe for keeping in a pump dispenser bottle next to the basin in the bathroom or the en suite; much nicer than a slimy bar of soap. It contains mild but effective foaming agents that cleanse and soften the skin. The fresh, herby notes of basil combined with the mint water, as well as the rosemary in the infusion, are excellent at removing any strong odour from the hands, and will leave you feeling sparkling clean and revived.

Makes approx. 200ml (7fl oz)

INGREDIENTS
80ml (5½ tbsp) Plantapon LGC
10ml (2 tsp) Lamesoft PO 65
10ml (2 tsp) rosemary-infused
  glycerine
100ml (6¾ tbsp) mint water
20 drops basil essential oil
40 drops grapefruit seed extract
  (as a preservative)

SPECIAL EQUIPMENT
thermometer
bottle with pump dispenser

SAFE STORAGE
Store in a cool, dry place away
from sunlight. Keeps for up to
3 months.

HOW TO APPLY
Pump a generous amount into the palms
of the hands and massage over wet hands
or body to create a good lather. Rinse
thoroughly. Follow with an application of
hand cream or body lotion.

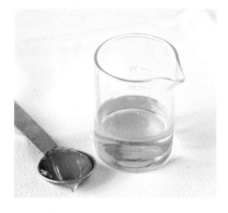

Step 1

Mix the Plantapon LGC and Lamesoft PO 65 together in a jug or beaker. Add the glycerine infusion (see page 37 for instructions on making an infusion), then set aside.

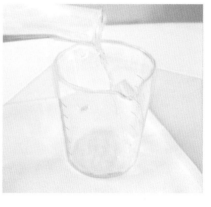

Step 2

Pour the mint water into a second, heatproof jug. Place the jug in a pan of simmering water and heat to 70–80°C (158–176°F). Maintain this temperature for 30 minutes, then remove from the heat.

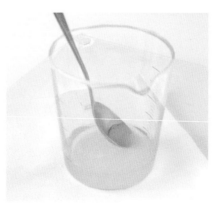

Step 3

Allow to cool, then combine the mint water with the Plantapon and Lamesoft mix, stirring slowly to avoid adding too much air and creating foam.

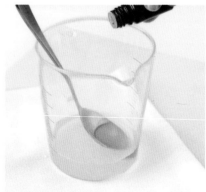

Step 4

Add the basil oil and preservative. Pour into a sterilized bottle, ideally with a pump dispenser. Label with the date and ingredients used.

Gardener's and Cook's Hand Scrub

Citrus fruits and salt have obvious associations with the kitchen. Lemon and orange have long been known as natural cleansing ingredients, and are incorporated here as zest. This yellowy-orange scrub will exfoliate and moisturize the hands in one treatment. The addition of the natural emulsifier Olivem 1000 means that the scrub will disperse well in warm water.

Makes approx. 100ml (3½fl oz)

INGREDIENTS
zest of 1 lemon and 1 orange
   (about 1g/¼ tsp in total)
30g (1oz) fine sea salt
28ml (5½ tsp) fractionated
   coconut oil
30ml (2 tbsp) sweet almond
   oil
10g (¼oz) Olivem 1000
5 drops grapefruit essential oil
5 drops lime essential oil

SPECIAL EQUIPMENT
chopping board
grater
small heatproof dish
coffee grinder
thermometer
small pestle and mortar

SAFE STORAGE
Store in a cool, dry place away
from sunlight. Keeps for up to
6 months.

HOW TO APPLY
Gently massage the scrub into dry hands,
paying special attention to the nails and
cuticles. Rinse thoroughly, then dry hands
and apply cream or lotion.

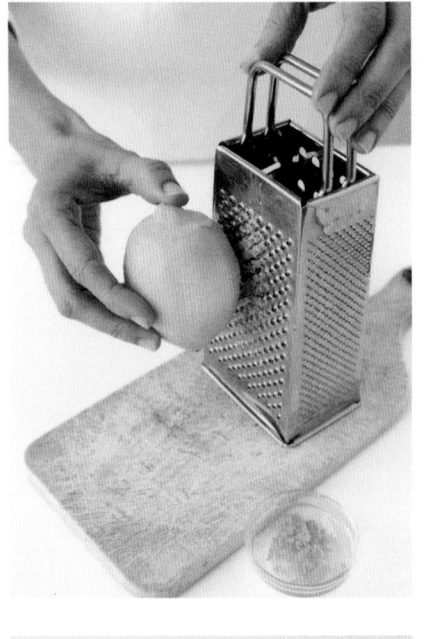

Step 1

Over a chopping board, zest the orange and the lemon using the fine side of a grater. Place the zest in a small heatproof dish in an oven heated to 100°C (212°F) to dry; this should take about 20 minutes. Grind the sea salt to a fine texture in a coffee grinder (unless you already have very fine salt). This should only take a few seconds. Then measure the fractionated coconut and sweet almond oils and Olivem 1000 into a heatproof jug. Place the jug in a pan of simmering water, and heat until the ingredients are dissolved.

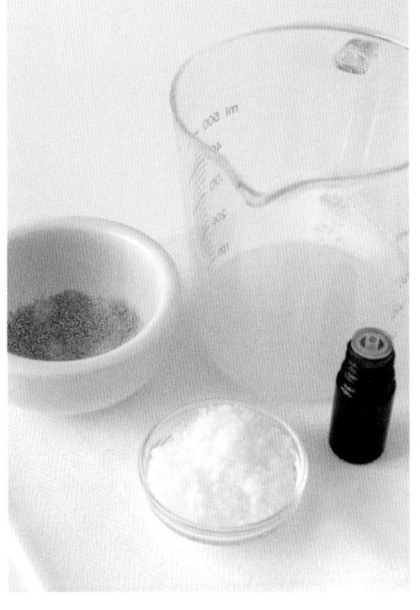

Step 2

Remove the dry zest from the oven, and grind using a pestle and mortar until you have a fine powder. Once the Olivem 1000 in the jug is dissolved in the oils, remove from the heat and cool slightly to below 50°C (122°F). Add the salt, dried zest and essential oils, and stir to mix. Continue to stir the mixture as it begins to cool and set, so that the salt and oils are combined together well and the mix is uniform. Spoon into a sterilized, airtight jar. Label with the date and ingredients used.

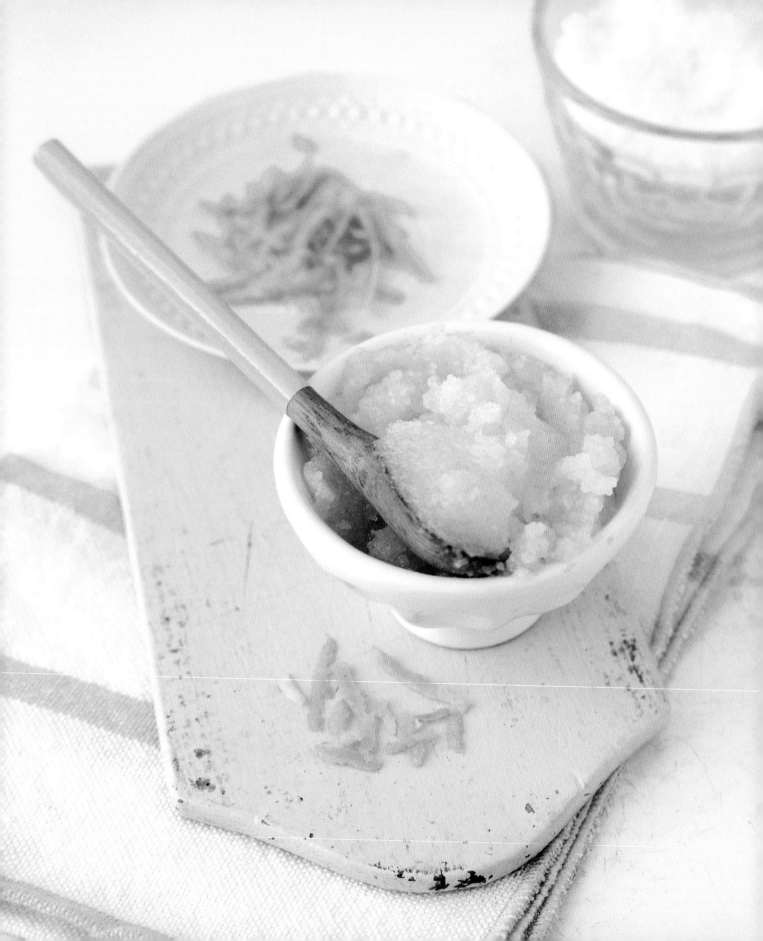

Nail Buffer

We would all love to have beautiful nails. Our hands are always on show, and we want them to look good. A shiny, smooth nail plate with healthy cuticles is the goal, especially if you find manicures hard to maintain or aren't a fan of nail varnish. This simple recipe can be made in a single jug, yet it's a real treat for the hands. You will be amazed at how polished and glossy your nails look after a few applications, so make sure you use the buffer regularly. We have suggested using tin oxide as the scrub ingredient; it can be obtained from pottery suppliers, but finely powdered pumice works equally well and can be sourced from online suppliers of cosmetic ingredients.

Makes approx. 50g (1¾oz)

INGREDIENTS
28ml (5½ tsp) sweet almond oil
2g (½ tsp) shea butter
5g (1 tsp) beeswax white BP
15g (½oz) tin oxide or very finely
  ground pumice
3 drops rosemary essential oil

SPECIAL EQUIPMENT
No special equipment required.

SAFE STORAGE
Store in a cool, dry place away from sunlight. Keeps for up to 12 months.

HOW TO APPLY
Using a cotton wool ball, massage a pea-sized amount of product firmly over the nails and cuticles, working all around the nail edges. Buff off the excess with clean cotton wool and repeat until you achieve the desired shine. Work under the nail and around the cuticle with an orange stick or cotton bud to remove any dirt and stains. Wash your hands to remove excess buffer.

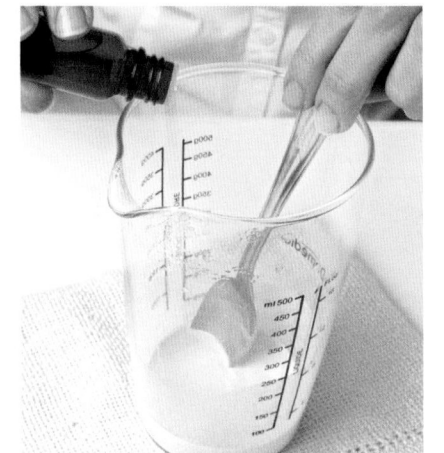

Step 1
Weigh all the ingredients except the tin oxide and rosemary oil into a heatproof jug. Place the jug in a pan of simmering water and heat until the beeswax is completely molten.

Step 2
Remove the jug from the heat and allow the mixture to cool slightly, but not so much that it solidifies. Once cooled, add the tin oxide and rosemary oil, and stir thoroughly to mix.

Step 3
Pour the mixture into small sterilized, airtight pots or tins. Label with the date and ingredients used. The recipe should make several small pots – enough for you and some friends.

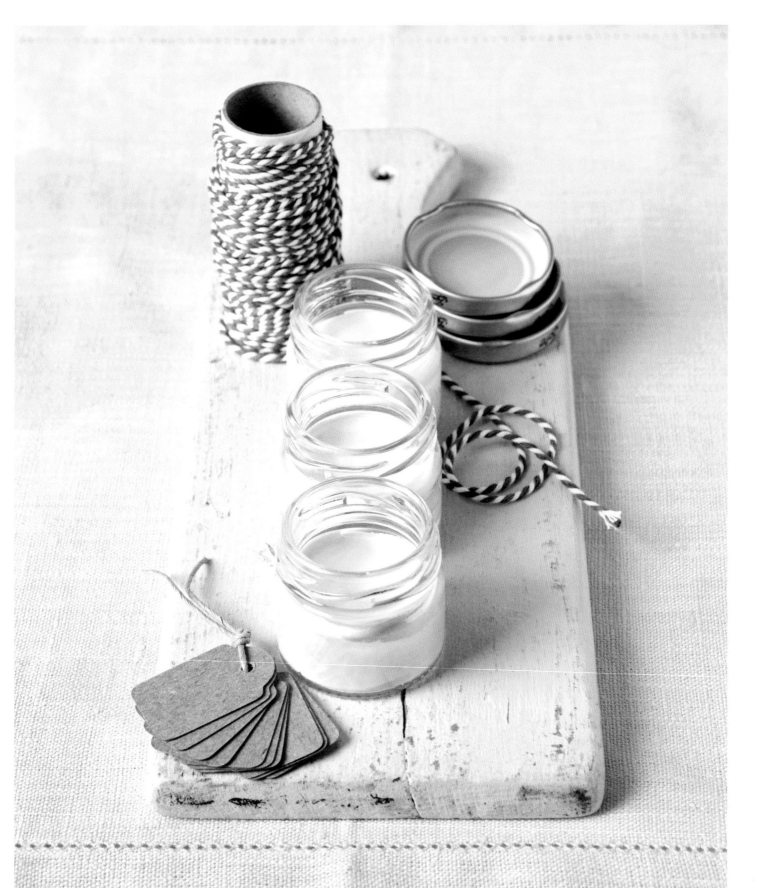

Hard-Working Hands Cream with Cinnamon, Geranium and Frankincense

If you are a gardener, work outside a lot or just have really dry skin, this aromatic hand cream is the perfect quick fix. The formulation contains nourishing oils and glycerine in sufficient quantities to impart a moisturizing film to the skin and help to protect against harsh conditions.

Makes approx. 100g (3½oz)

INGREDIENTS
Phase 1
7g (1½ tsp) Emulsifying Wax BP
8ml (1½ tsp) grapeseed oil
50ml (3½ tbsp) rose water
20ml (4 tsp) spring water
2.5ml (½ tsp) glycerine

Phase 2
1ml (¼ tsp) vitamin E oil
  in dilution
5ml (1 tsp) rosehip oil
4ml (¾ tsp) jojoba oil

2 drops cinnamon leaf essential oil
3 drops geranium essential oil
2 drops frankincense essential oil
20 drops grapefruit seed extract
  (as a preservative)

SPECIAL EQUIPMENT
thermometer
stick blender or milk frother

SAFE STORAGE
Store in a cool, dry place away from sunlight. Keeps for up to 3 months.

HOW TO APPLY
Rub a small amount into the hands and massage gently into the cuticles, allowing the oils to be absorbed.

Tip!
Because the formulation is so rich, this cream is especially good for winter use and, as such, we often make it as a Christmas gift. The spicy frankincense and cinnamon leaf essential oils give a warm and comforting fragrance, and make it even more festive!

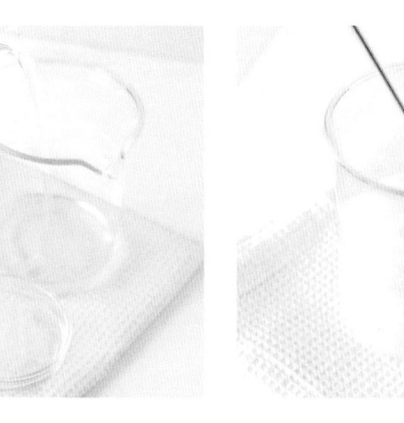

Step 1
Measure the Phase 1 ingredients into a heatproof jug. Place the jug in a pan of simmering water and heat to 75–80°C (167–176°F). Maintain this temperature for 30 minutes.

Step 2
Remove from the heat and cool to around 50°C (122°F), then whizz with a stick blender or milk frother until emulsified. Allow to de-aerate, then cool the mixture to around 40°C (104°F).

Step 3
Add the vitamin E, rosehip and jojoba oils with the essential oils and preservative. Stir to mix thoroughly, then pour into a sterilized, airtight jar. Label with the date and ingredients used.

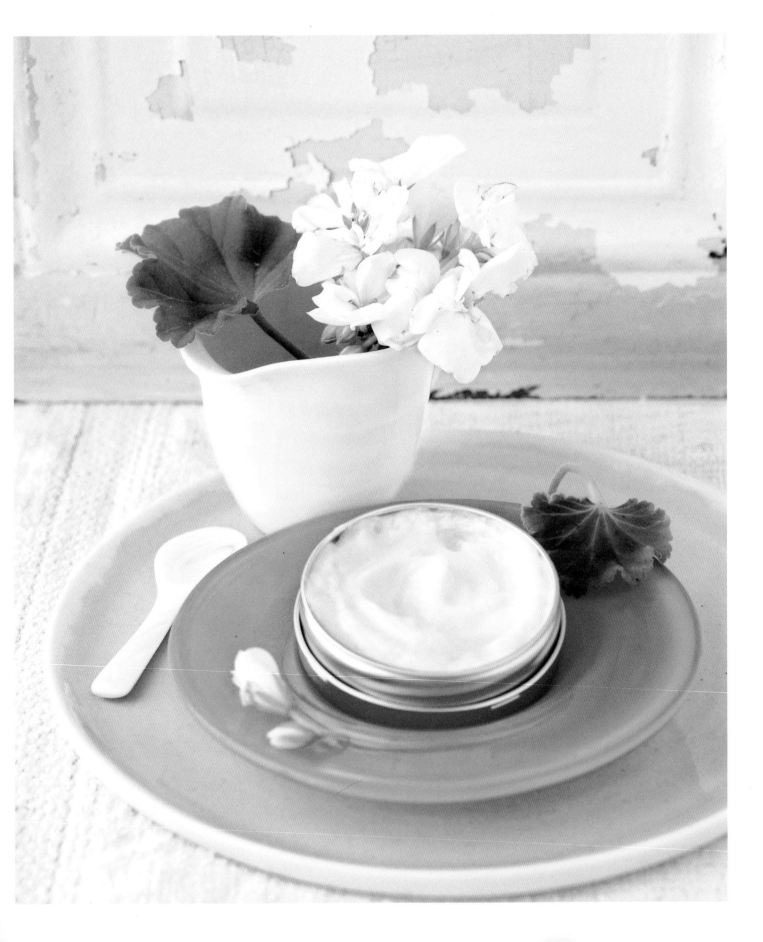

Fit Feet Foot Soak

Wake up tired feet with this deodorizing foot soak. It can be crafted very quickly from ingredients that may well already be in your larder or bathroom cabinet. Epsom salts are easily obtainable from a pharmacy or health-food store. You'll find them invaluable as an inexpensive yet effective detoxifying bath soak ingredient in their own right. Tea tree oil is renowned for its antimicrobial qualities.

Makes approx. 100g (3½ oz)

INGREDIENTS
5g (1 tsp) unperfumed soap
5g (1 tsp) dried lavender flowers
65g (2¼oz) oat flour or porridge
   oats
5g (1 tsp) shea butter
10g (¼oz) Epsom salts
10g (¼oz) sodium bicarbonate
   (baking soda)
4 drops tea tree essential oil
4 drops peppermint essential oil
2 drops lavender essential oil

SPECIAL EQUIPMENT
chopping board
grater
coffee grinder

SAFE STORAGE
Store in a cool, dry place away from sunlight. Keeps for up to 3 months.

HOW TO USE
Sprinkle a generous handful of the soak into a bowl of warm water and stir to dissolve. Rest your feet in the water for 5–10 minutes, or as long as you like. Your feet should feel revived and softer for the relaxing experience. Dry the feet thoroughly. To complete the restorative treat, apply a rich cream or massage oil.

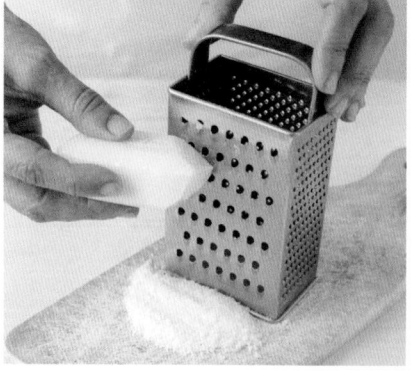

Step 1
Over a chopping board, grate the soap using the coarse side of a grater. The soap in the soak will not only cleanse the skin, but also help to disperse the oils.

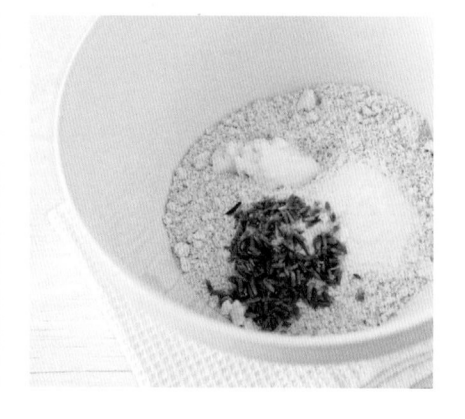

Step 2
Weigh the lavender flowers, oat flour, shea butter and grated soap into a bowl. If you don't have specialist oat flour, simply use porridge oats.

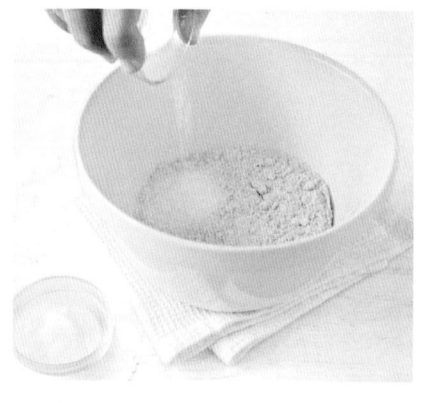

Step 3
Transfer the mixture into a coffee grinder (it should just about fit in one go), and blitz until the ingredients are reduced to a fine powder. Return to the bowl, and add the Epsom salts and sodium bicarbonate (baking soda) to the powder.

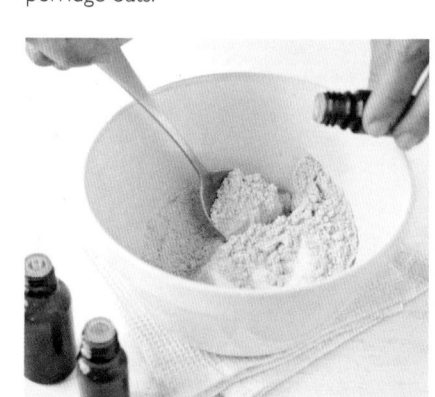

Step 4
Finally, add the essential oils to the powder. Stir to mix completely, and pour into a sterilized, airtight jar or bottle. Label with the date and ingredients used. The recipe amount should be sufficient for several soaks.

Adaptation:

Fizzing Foot Soak

....

The addition of citric acid to this recipe reacts with the sodium bicarbonate (baking soda) to create the fizz.

Makes approx. 100g (3½oz)

INGREDIENTS

5g (1 tsp) unperfumed soap
55g (2oz) oat flour or porridge oats
5g (1 tsp) shea butter
10g (¼oz) citric acid
10g (¼oz) Epsom salts
15g (½oz) sodium bicarbonate (baking soda)
4 drops tea tree essential oil
4 drops peppermint essential oil
2 drops lavender essential oil

Ensure that all equipment is completely dry to avoid any moisture coming into contact with the mixture and starting a fizzing reaction. Grate the soap, then weigh the oat flour (or porridge oats), shea butter and soap into a bowl. Reduce the mixture to a fine powder in a coffee grinder and return to the bowl. Add the citric acid, Epsom salts, sodium bicarbonate (baking soda) and essential oils, then stir to mix and pour into a sterilized, airtight jar. Label with the date and ingredients used.

SAFE STORAGE
Store in a cool, dry place away from sunlight. Keeps for up to 3 months.

....

HOW TO USE
See the Fit Feet Foot Soak (opposite). The soak will start to fizz as soon as it is immersed in water.

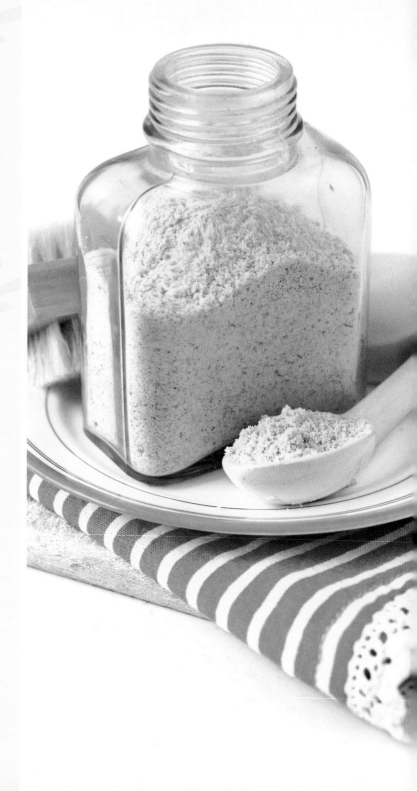

Foot Refresher Spray

Are your feet making you feel frazzled? Our zingy foot-spray recipe is such a breeze to make, you can even mix it in the bottle. It contains a bathroom-cabinet favourite, witch hazel, well known for its ability to soothe insect bites on account of its astringent and cooling effect. Aching, puffy feet will instantly feel the benefit of the refreshing spray; it evaporates speedily on the skin, and you can use it as often as required throughout the day. Why not also try spritzing the liquid directly into summer sandals and trainers to refresh them with the minty scent.

Makes approx. 50ml (1 ½fl oz)

INGREDIENTS
50ml (3½ tbsp) distilled witch hazel BPC
2 drops each of peppermint, lemon, cypress and lavender essential oils

SPECIAL EQUIPMENT
spray bottle with cap

SAFE STORAGE
Store in a cool, dry place away from sunlight. Keeps for up to 3 months.

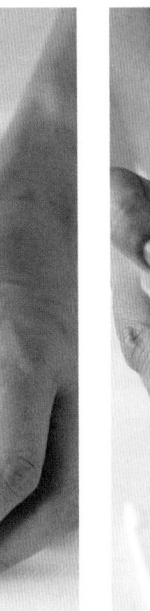

Step 1
Pour the witch hazel into a sterilized glass or plastic spray bottle. You could also fill an additional small bottle for your handbag.

Step 2
Add the essential oils. Secure the cap on the bottle and shake to mix. Label with the date and ingredients used.

Adaptation:
Fit Feet Foot Spray

This variation on the Foot Refresher Spray contains antimicrobial oils of tea tree and eucalyptus to help keep your feet smelling sweet.

Makes approx. 50ml (1 ½fl oz)

INGREDIENTS
50ml (3½ tbsp) distilled witch hazel BPC
2 drops each of tea tree, eucalyptus and lavender essential oils

See the Foot Refresher Spray for method and application.

SAFE STORAGE
Store in a cool, dry place away from sunlight. Keeps for up to 3 months.

HOW TO APPLY
Spray liberally over tired feet. Briefly allow to dry if you're putting your shoes back on.

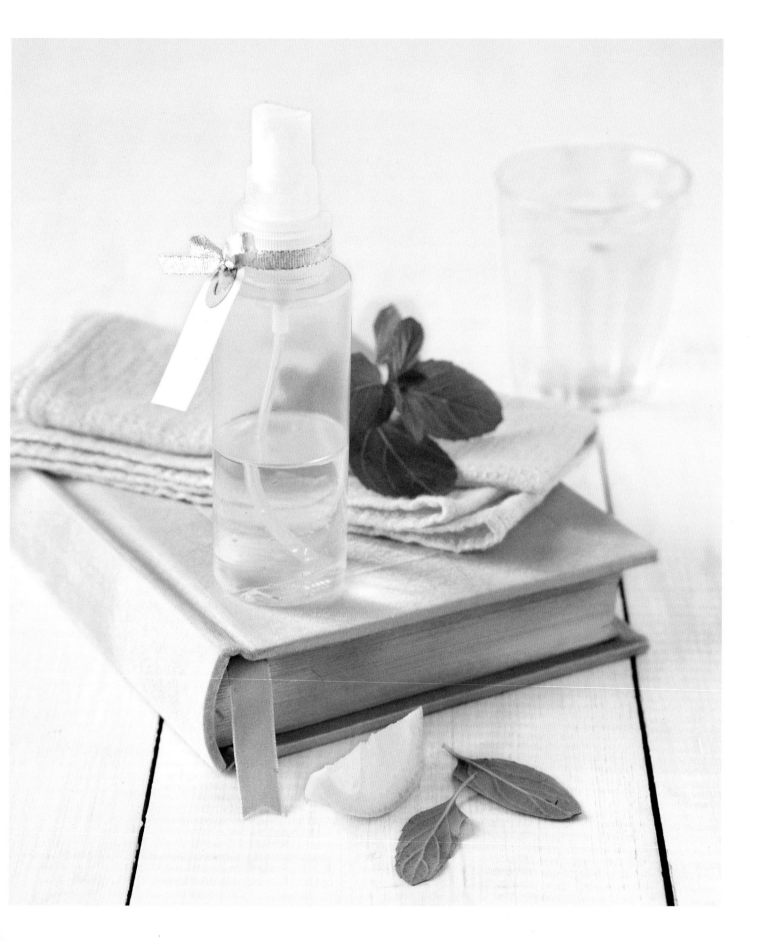

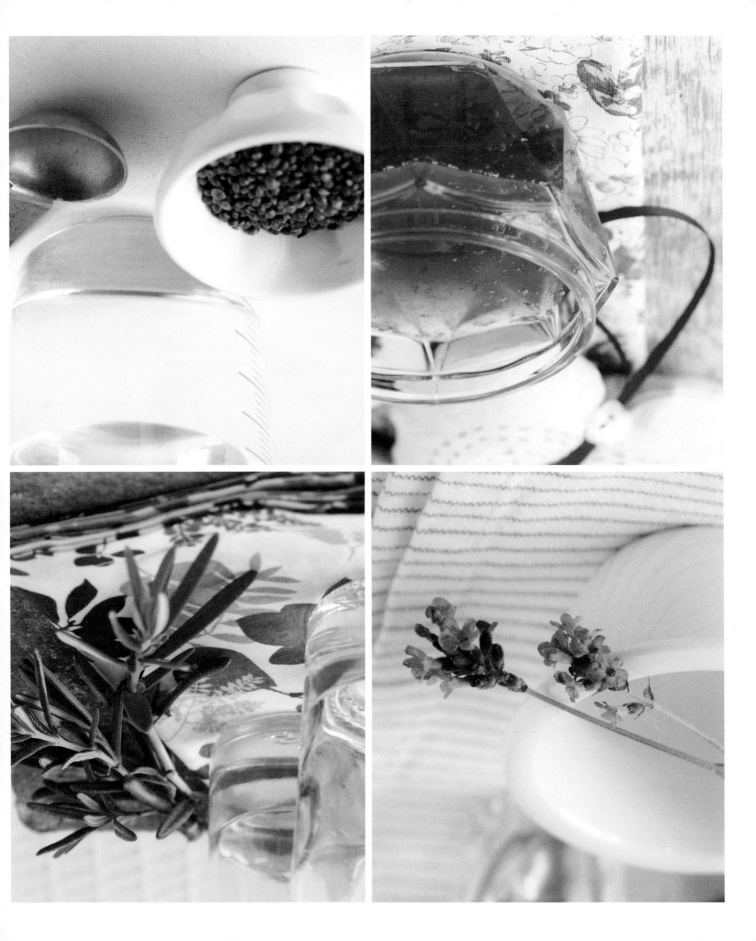

HAIR

Beer Shandy Shampoo with Lime Oil

Beer has been adopted as a hair treatment for generations; its ability to add gloss to and condition the hair was known to our mothers and grandmothers. It contains protein and nutrients, which help to protect and volumize the hair, as well as enhance shine. For this recipe, we like to use a craft-style beer from a small brewery, rather than canned lager, as we believe it produces a better result. Don't be put off by the thought of smelling of beer: the lime essential oil gives a zesty, clean freshness to the hair.

Makes approx. 100ml (3½fl oz)

INGREDIENTS
40ml (2¾ tbsp) Plantapon LGC
5ml (1 tsp) Lamesoft PO 65
5ml (1 tsp) rosemary-infused
    glycerine
50ml (3½ tbsp) beer or lager
    (any good craft beer)
10 drops lime essential oil
20 drops grapefruit seed extract
    (as a preservative)

SPECIAL EQUIPMENT
thermometer

SAFE STORAGE
Store in a cool, dry place away from sunlight. Keeps for up to 3 months.

HOW TO APPLY
This shampoo contains mild but effective cleansing agents, and is suitable for all hair types.

Apply to wet hair and massage in gently to generate foam. Rinse out well. If you wish, follow with a conditioner suited to your hair type. To continue with the beer theme, you could try the Hair Rinse on page 129, either massaged in directly after shampooing or spritzed on to towel-dried hair.

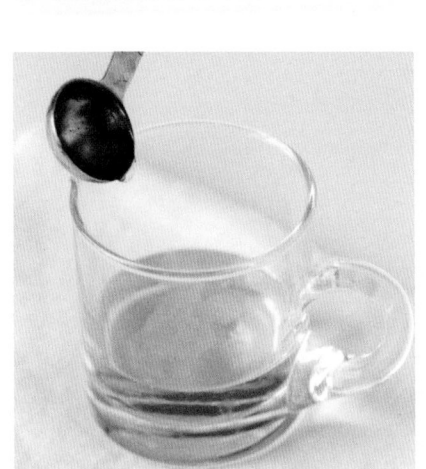

Step 1
Mix the Plantapon LGC and Lamesoft PO 65 together in a jug or beaker. Add the glycerine infusion (see page 37 for instructions), then set aside. Pour the beer into a second, heatproof jug.

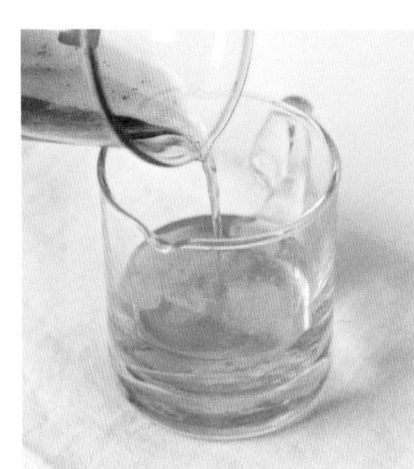

Step 2
Place the jug with the beer in a pan of simmering water and heat to 70–80°C (158–176°F) for 30 minutes. Remove from the heat and allow to cool. Add the beer to the Plantapon and Lamesoft mix.

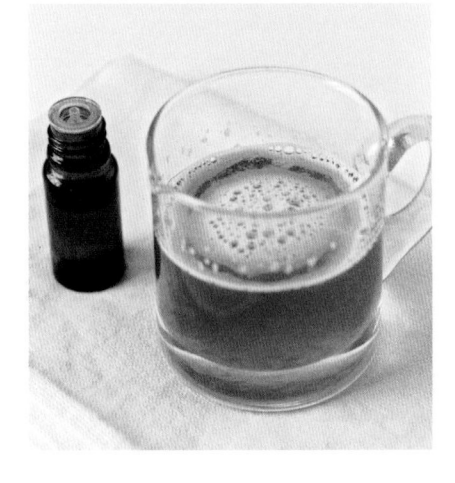

Step 3
Stir the mix slowly to avoid adding too much air and creating foam. Add the lime oil and preservative. Pour into a sterilized bottle with a cap. Label with the date and ingredients used.

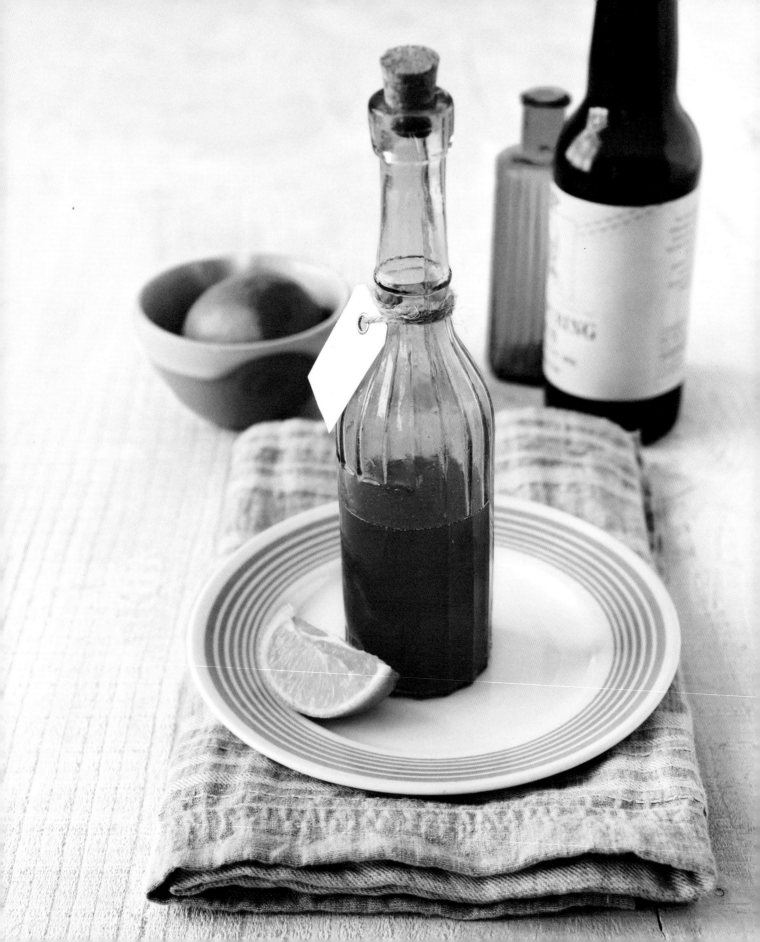

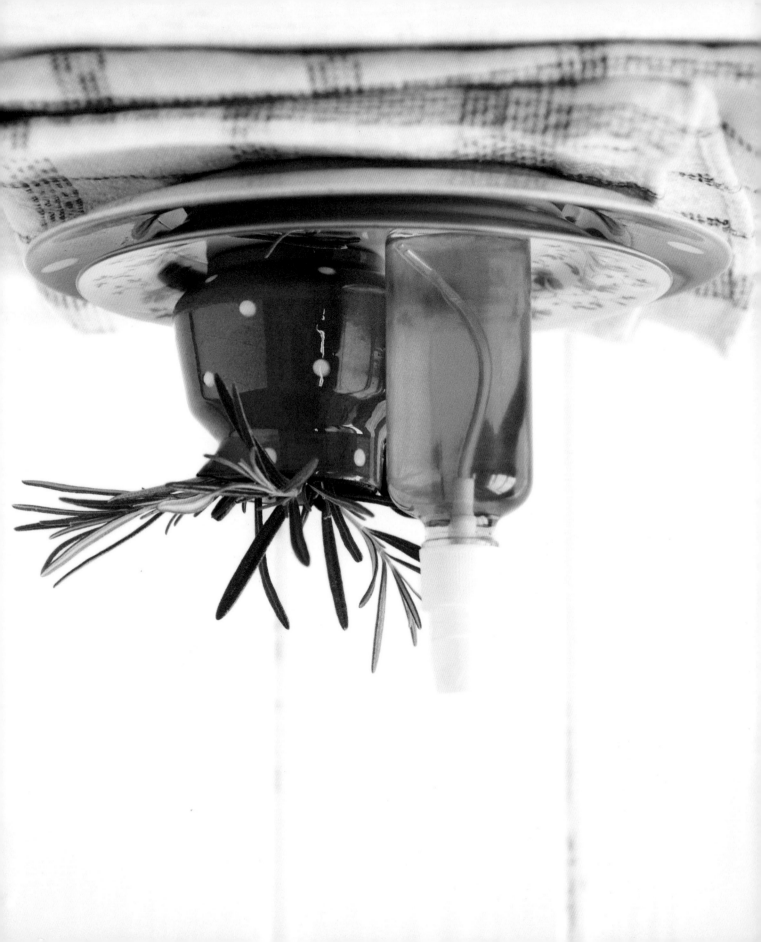

Hair Rinse with Beer, Lemon and Rosemary

Makes approx. 100ml (3½fl oz)

INGREDIENTS
10ml (2 tsp) fresh lemon
  juice
40ml (2¾ tbsp) beer (any
  good craft beer)
38ml (2½ tbsp) water
10ml (2 tsp) cider vinegar
5 drops rosemary essential oil
5 drops lemon essential oil
20 drops grapefruit seed
  extract (as a preservative)

SPECIAL EQUIPMENT
lemon squeezer
thermometer
funnel
spray bottle with cap (if using
  as a conditioning spray)

SAFE STORAGE
Store in a cool, dry place away
from sunlight. Keeps for up to
3 months.

Our hair rinse is another recipe that makes use of beer for its well-known haircare benefits. The protein in beer helps to strengthen and nourish the hair, and also assists the repair of hair damaged by blow-drying and straighteners. A simple blend of kitchen ingredients, the recipe provides a traditional-style rinse for brightness and shine. Because it contains water, a preservative is required. The addition of lemon and rosemary essential oils gives a fresh, herbal fragrance to the product and a light scent to the hair on application. The rinse can be used after shampooing, either massaged in and left, or applied with a spray mister.

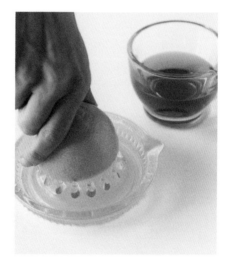

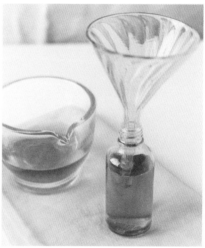

HOW TO APPLY
After shampooing, pour sufficient rinse on to the hair to coat it, and massage well. No rinsing is required.

Tip!
This recipe is also ideal to use as a conditioning spray, which can be misted on to the hair from a fine-spray bottle. Simply spray on to clean, towel-dried hair and comb through gently to remove any tangles. Again, there's no need to rinse off. Style and dry your hair as usual.

Step 1

Squeeze a lemon and separate the juice, making sure you remove any pips. Measure the beer, water, cider vinegar and freshly squeezed lemon juice into a heatproof jug. Place the jug in a pan of simmering water and heat to 80°C (176°F). Maintain this temperature for 30 minutes to ensure that the resulting liquid is sufficiently sterile.

Step 2

Remove from the heat and allow to cool to about 40°C (104°F). Add the essential oils and preservative, and stir thoroughly to mix. The recipe should be brown in colour, although this will depend on the beer used. Pour through a funnel into a sterilized screw-topped bottle for use as a rinse. Label with the date and ingredients used.

Anti-Dandruff Scalp Massage Lotion

There is a long-standing tradition of using rosemary and lavender in haircare. Rosemary, in particular, helps to stimulate the scalp and assists hair growth. Lavender is renowned for its calming properties, and can help to soothe a dry, itchy scalp. This fresh recipe can be crafted in a matter of minutes; it should be used straight away, rather than stored (although any remaining lotion will keep in the fridge for a few days). The addition of vodka to the water allows the essential oils to mix well into the solution, so it won't leave the scalp or hair feeling greasy.

Rather surprisingly, the recipe also makes a great eau de toilette; see our suggestions below for some more wonderfully aromatic essential oil combinations to blend with the water and alcohol.

Makes approx. 20ml (¾fl oz)

INGREDIENTS
1 tsp vodka
1 tbsp water
3 drops rosemary essential oil
5 drops lavender essential oil

SPECIAL EQUIPMENT
No special equipment required.

SAFE STORAGE
Make and use fresh. Keeps for up to 3 days when stored in the fridge.

HOW TO APPLY
Massage gently into the scalp and leave on. Use regularly to maintain scalp health.

Tip!
For an alternative fresh eau de toilette, combine rosemary and lavender oils with lemon, orange and spearmint. For a zesty scent, try lime, bergamot or grapefruit with sweet orange and neroli. For something more sensual, mix ylang-ylang with jasmine and frankincense or cedarwood.

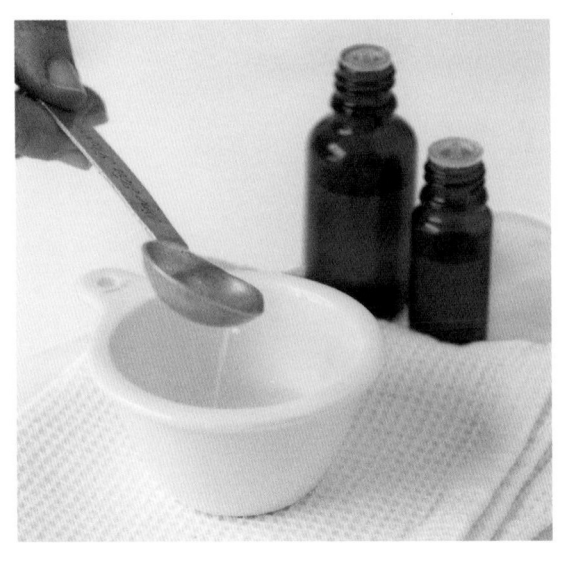

Step 1
Measure all the ingredients into a small beaker or jug. Alternatively, if you're not going to use all the lotion in a single application, you could measure the ingredients straight into a small bottle, ready to store in the fridge after the first use. Using measuring spoons makes this really quick work.

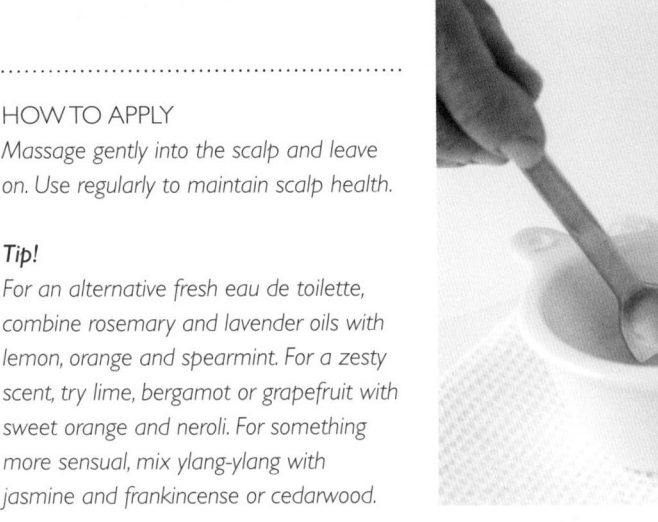

Step 2
The vodka, water and essential oils will mix together very easily, but it is advisable to stir or shake the mixture to ensure the oils are well incorporated before use. Apply the lotion immediately to the scalp.

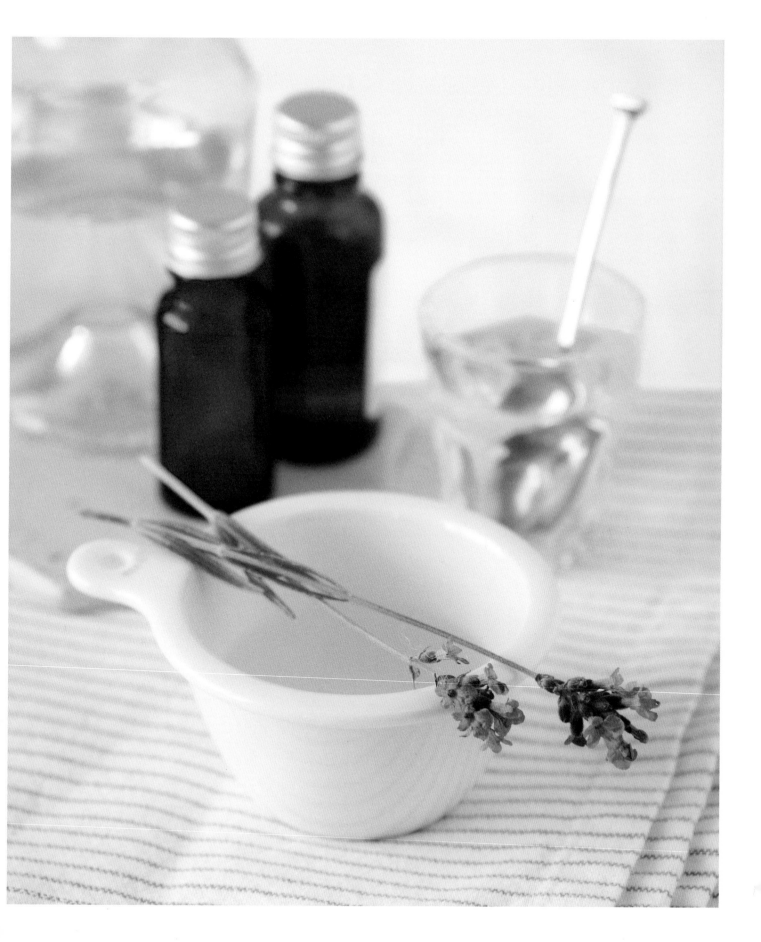

Invigorating Scalp Massage Oil *(for greasy hair)*

The peppermint, rosemary and eucalyptus essential oils in this massage oil are great for stimulating the scalp. Super-quick and easy to make, the recipe also contains a blend of nourishing oils and no water, so a preservative is not required. The oil stores well, and the quantity should be sufficient for several applications.

Makes approx. 50ml (1½fl oz)

INGREDIENTS
20ml (4 tsp) jojoba oil
15ml (3 tsp) evening
 primrose oil
15ml (3 tsp) borage oil
4 drops peppermint essential oil
3 drops rosemary essential oil
3 drops eucalyptus essential oil

SPECIAL EQUIPMENT
optional: funnel

SAFE STORAGE
Store in a cool, dry place away from sunlight. Keeps for up to 6 months.

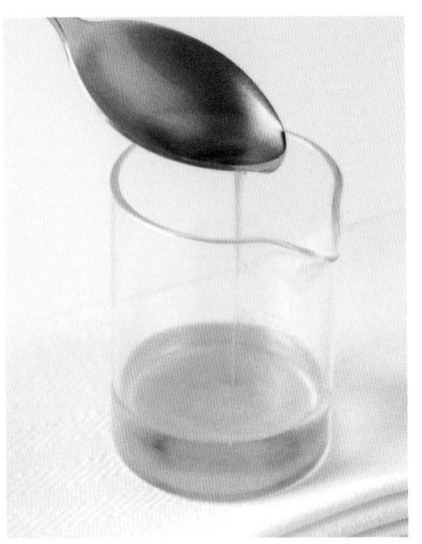

Step 1
Measure all the ingredients into a small glass beaker or jug, and stir with a stainless steel teaspoon to mix thoroughly.

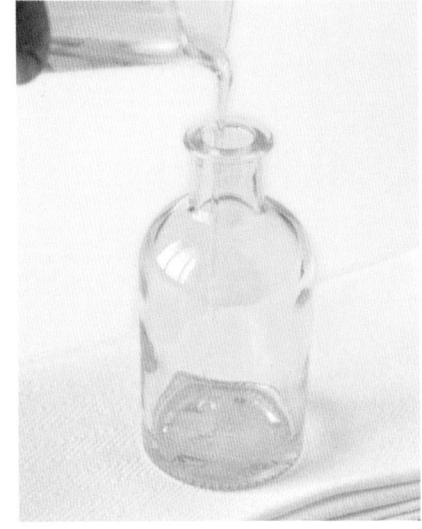

Step 2
Pour the oil into a sterilized, airtight glass bottle. A small funnel may help the transfer. Label with the date and ingredients used.

Adaptation:
Nourishing Scalp Massage Oil (for dry hair)

This adaptation uses a rich blend of botanical oils, combined with soothing essential oils, to create a moisturizing scalp treatment.

Makes approx. 50ml (1½fl oz)

INGREDIENTS
20ml (4 tsp) jojoba oil
15ml (3 tsp) evening primrose oil
15ml (3 tsp) rosehip oil
4 drops lavender essential oil
3 drops geranium essential oil
3 drops camomile essential oil
 in dilution

See the Invigorating Scalp Massage Oil for method and application.

SAFE STORAGE
Store in a cool, dry place away from sunlight. Keeps for up to 6 months.

HOW TO APPLY
Massage gently into the scalp, and leave on for about 30 minutes. Remove by washing hair with your chosen shampoo. Use regularly to maintain scalp health.

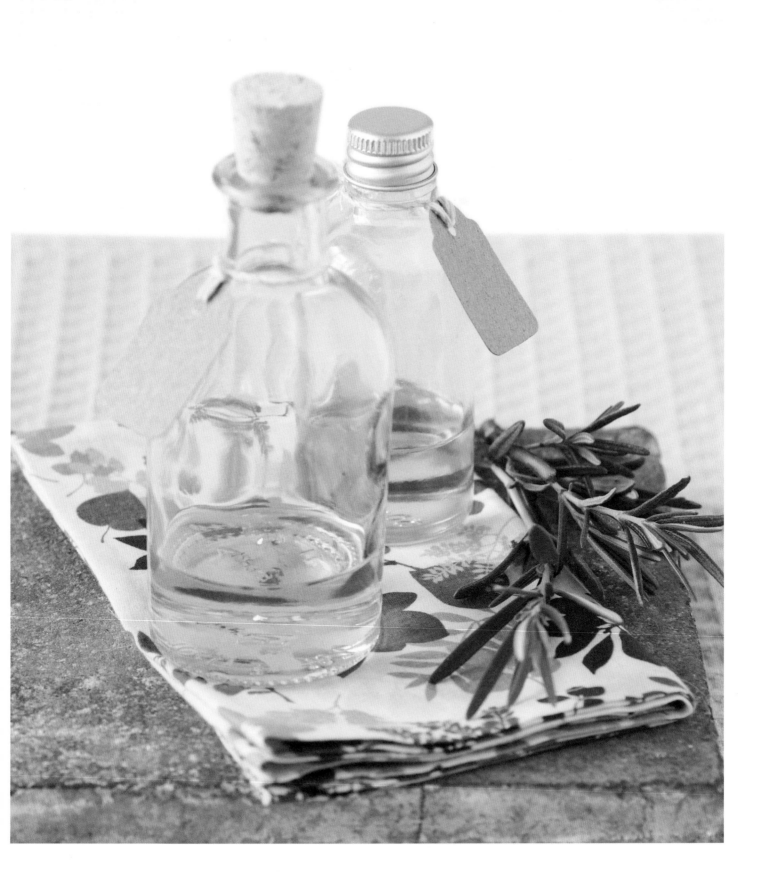

Linseed Anti-Frizz Styling Gel

Based on nourishing linseeds, this fast-drying styling gel moisturizes hair and defines curls without stiffness or crunchiness. Very simple to create and using only a couple of inexpensive store-cupboard ingredients, it's a recipe that deserves to be tried out by anyone with hard-to-tame wavy or curly hair.

Makes approx. 500ml (17fl oz)

INGREDIENTS
2 tbsp linseeds (flaxseeds)
500ml (17fl oz) spring water
optional: 20 drops grapefruit seed
    extract (as a preservative) per
    100ml (3½fl oz)

SPECIAL EQUIPMENT
thermometer
sieve (sifter)
large jug

SAFE STORAGE
If you do not add a preservative, make and use fresh. Keeps for up to 3 days when stored in the fridge. Otherwise, store in a cool, dry place away from sunlight. Keeps for up to 3 months.

HOW TO APPLY
After shampooing, apply the gel to damp hair and either leave to dry naturally or blow-dry hair using a diffuser.

Tip!
You can also dilute the gel to use as a sprayable version, in which case you will need to ensure that you add additional preservative to the larger volume of liquid.

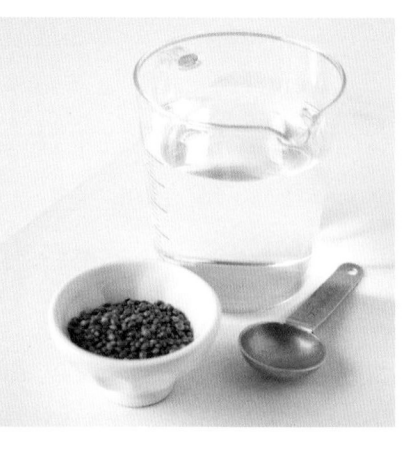

Step 1
Weigh out the linseeds (flaxseeds), and measure the water into a jug. Pour the linseeds and water into a pan, and heat to 70–80°C (158–176°F).

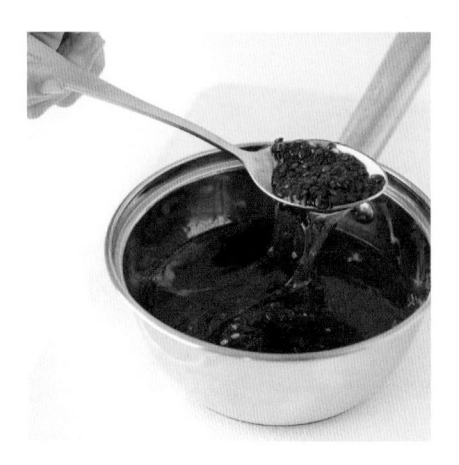

Step 2
Simmer for about 30 minutes. The mixture will thicken and gain an increasingly gel-like consistency the longer you leave it, but this varies depending on the seeds' freshness.

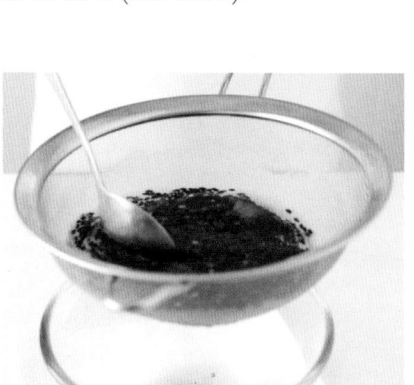

Step 3
Pour the mixture into a sieve (sifter) and allow the gel to drip into a bowl, leaving behind the linseed husks. You can use a spoon to push the gel through the sieve.

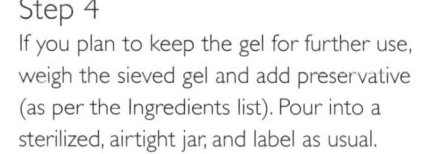

Step 4
If you plan to keep the gel for further use, weigh the sieved gel and add preservative (as per the Ingredients list). Pour into a sterilized, airtight jar, and label as usual.

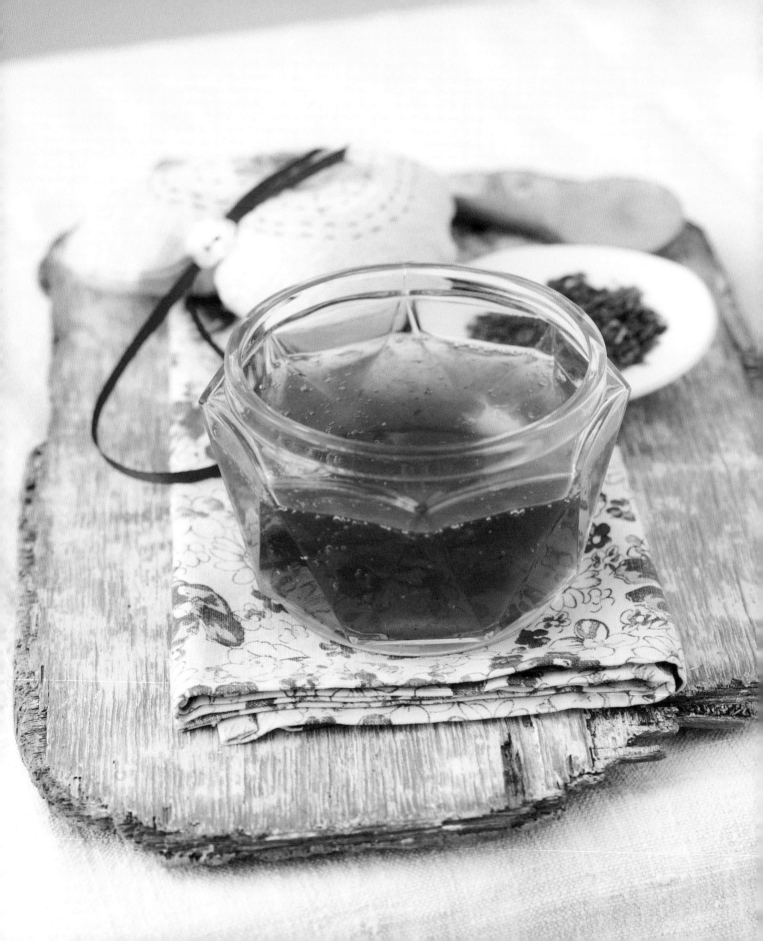

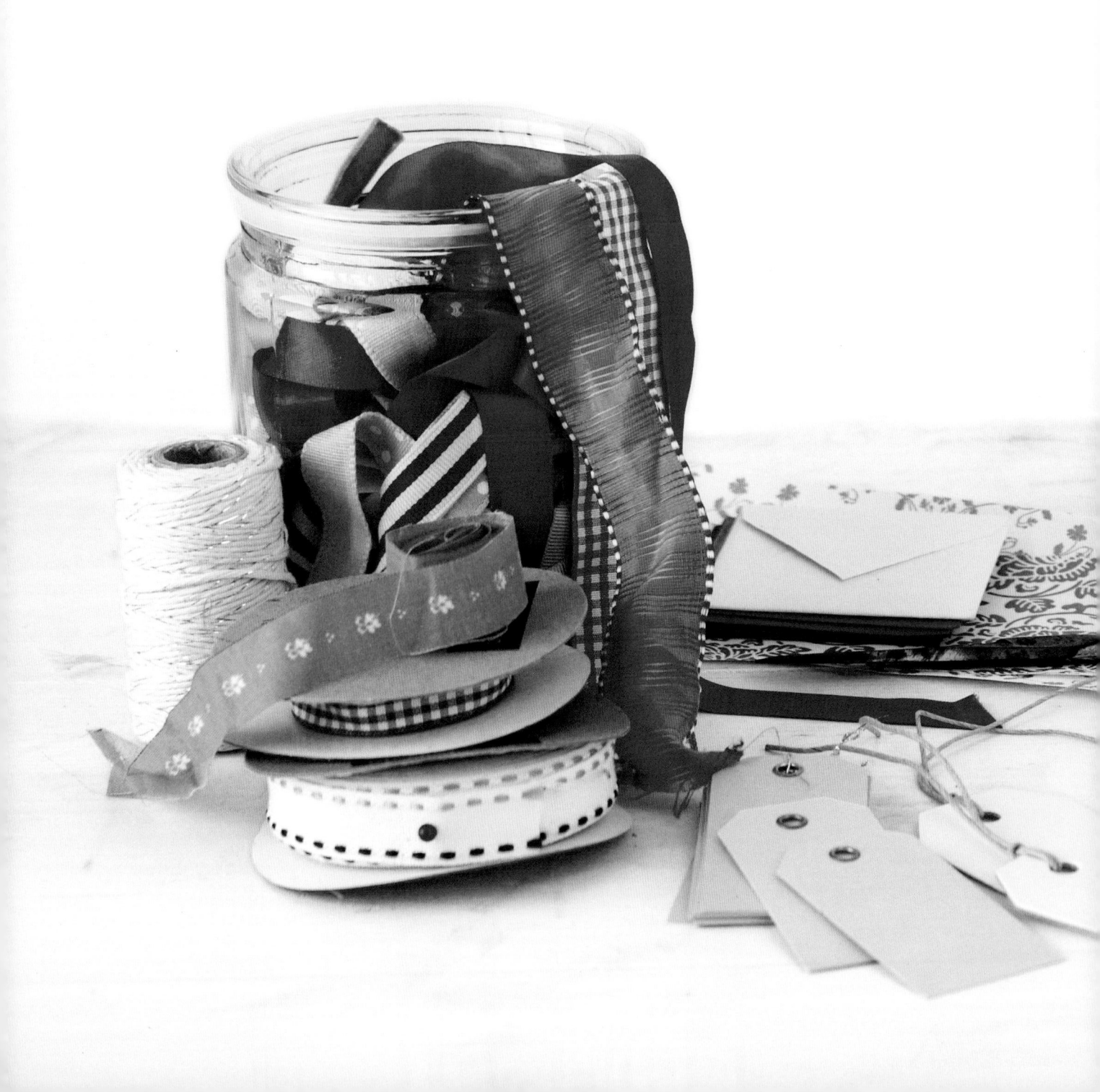

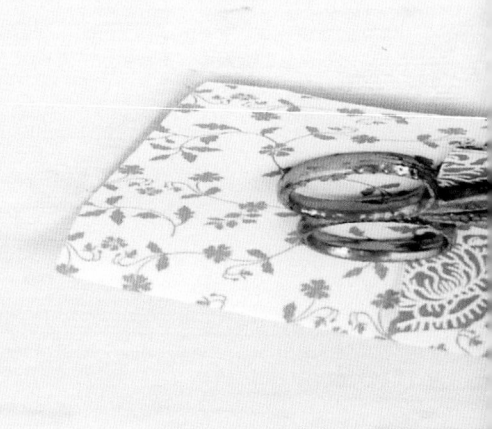

Finishing Touches

CREATING YOUR OWN BEAUTY RECIPES IS SUCH REWARDING WORK AND, HAVING LEARNED HOW TO MASTER MANY DIFFERENT PRODUCTS, YOU WILL OF COURSE WANT THEM TO LOOK THEIR BEST, WHETHER YOU DISPLAY THEM ON YOUR DRESSING TABLE OR BATHROOM SHELF, OR PRESENT THEM TO FRIENDS AND FAMILY. WE HAVE GATHERED TOGETHER A FEW TIPS AND INSPIRING IDEAS TO GIVE YOUR CREATIONS A LITTLE BIT OF STYLING MAGIC AND MAKE YOUR GIFTS EXTRA-SPECIAL. BUT THE REAL THRILL FOR THE RECIPIENTS WILL BE WHEN THEY ACTUALLY USE YOUR OWN HAND-CRAFTED BEAUTY PRODUCTS.

Adding the Finishing Touch

It doesn't matter whether you're giving your handmade products away or keeping them for yourself, you'll want them to look good. But remember: all cosmetics require the correct type of packaging, with container materials that suit the product inside, and lids that don't leak. As we've discussed in 'Containers and Storage' (see page 30), a face cream, for example, is generally better suited to a glass jar than a tin. You can buy functional, inexpensive containers online, but you can also repurpose some you already have.

BOTTLES AND JARS

- **Put to reuse:** Perhaps you have some lovely packaging from a premium skincare product you have finished that would be ideal for a home-made cream, or some fancy food jars that might suit a scrub or a body butter. Set aside Kilner jars and lever-top bottles for just these uses, as well as jam jars and glass bottles of varying sizes with their lids. Don't forget that they must be cleaned and sterilized before use.
- **Go vintage:** Search out vintage bottles that can be reused for lotions, toners or bath oils; try decorating the neck with a pretty ribbon. If you have any beads, charms or other small pieces of unused jewellery, tie them to the ribbon. Make a point of keeping ribbon or nice twine to attach gift tags or secure cellophane wrap (see below).

TINS, BOXES, BAGS AND WRAPPINGS

- **Tins:** Lidded tins are useful for dry products such as bath powders and foot soaks. For a home-made touch, stick a band of patterned wrapping paper around the outside of the tin. Attach a pretty scoop or vintage teaspoon to create a really attractive gift. Vintage tea caddies often have beautiful designs, but the tins may not be in pristine condition. You can still use them if you pour the powder into a plastic bag, seal it and then tuck it inside the tin.
- **Boxes:** If you've received anything in a gift box of the 'tray and push-on lid' style, you have something that you can instantly repurpose with the help of a strip of gift wrap stuck over the box. Wrap some coloured tissue

paper around the bottles or jars you place inside the box to prevent them getting damaged.
- **Paper bags:** Similarly, keep any premium small paper carrier bags with rope handles. Stick a photograph, postcard or repurposed greetings card image to each side to create a whole new gift bag.
- **Fabric bags:** Collect small fabric (frequently organza) bags with drawstrings, which are often given away, or indeed make your own very simple gift bags from printed cotton scraps. To work out the size of the piece of fabric required, check the height of the item, and allow extra for tying; then double the width measurement. Fold the fabric in half, and stitch along one side and the bottom. Turn the bag right side out and tie with a piece of ribbon. This would be ideal for products in bottles or jars.
- **Wrappings:** Bath bombs (see pages 96–99) need to be kept dry so that they don't start to fizz; put them in cellophane wrap. Cut a large circle or square of wrap; it needs to be considerably larger than the bath bomb itself to allow for a plume of cellophane at the top. Secure with an elastic band, then tie a ribbon over the band and finish with a bow. (You could also use decorative storage jars: simply place the bombs inside, ideally cushioned by packing straw, so they can be admired on a shelf.)

LABEL IT UP!

- **Labels:** Remember to mark each product with the ingredients used and the date it was made; this information can be hand-written on a home-made tag crafted from coloured card or a small luggage label tied to the gift. Embellish further by using rubber stamps and coloured ink pads to decorate tags and plain wrapping paper. Look for pretty self-adhesive labels in stationery stores, or check online sites that allow you to use templates to design and print off bespoke labels.
- **Envelopes:** If you're using a gift tag, a decorative envelope adds a stylish touch. Make your own from left-over wrapping paper: open out an envelope of the right size and adopt it as a template; fold and stick down the edges.

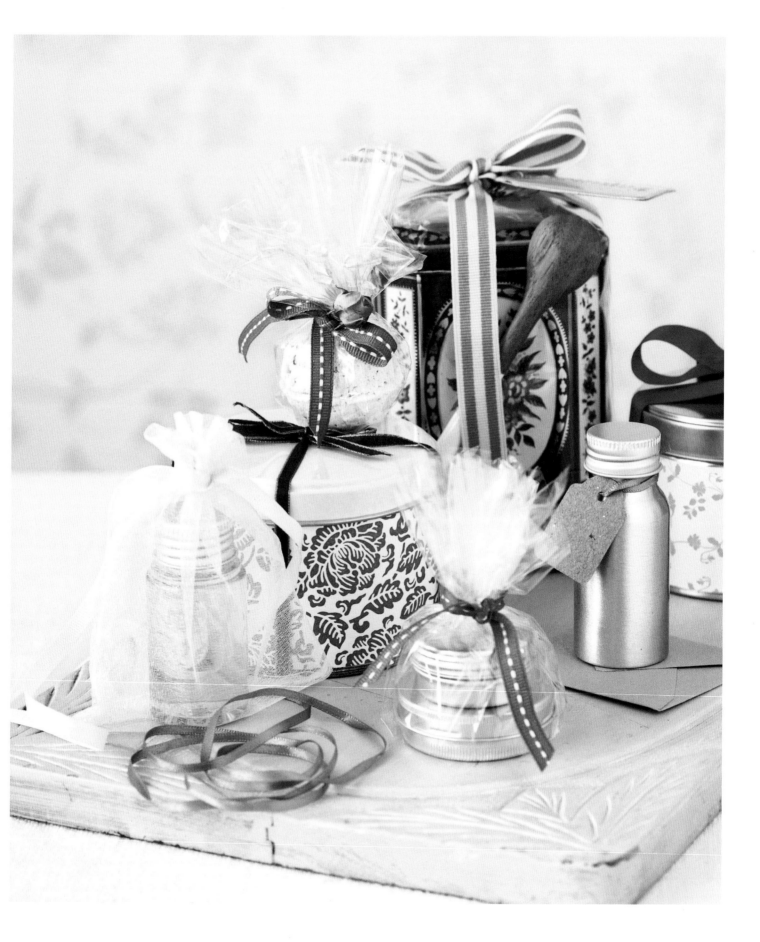

Glossary of Ingredients

This table includes all ingredients we have included in our recipes, listing their INCI name and their benefits when used in skin- or haircare. By law, the labels on all cosmetic and personal care products must contain a list of ingredients used. The cosmetics industry uses a common naming system known as the International Nomenclature for Cosmetic Ingredients (INCI). This means that the same ingredient names, based on scientific names, are used internationally; this helps people to avoid the ingredients to which they are allergic.

KEY:

The symbols indicate where you will be able to buy the ingredients featured in the recipes in this book:

✚ CHEMIST (DRUGSTORE)
◌ HEALTH-FOOD STORE
@ INTERNET
🛒 SUPERMARKET

COMMON NAME	INCI (EU) NAME	BENEFIT
ACAI BERRY JUICE ◌	EUTERPE OLERACEA FRUIT EXTRACT	Rich in vitamin C and antioxidants, which help to protect the skin by scavenging the harmful free radicals generated by UV and pollution, thus promoting a healthy, radiant complexion.
ALMOND EXTRACT FLAVOURING 🛒	NATURAL FLAVOURING, ETHANOL	Natural almond flavour for lip balms.
ALOE VERA JUICE ◌	ALOE BARBADENSIS LEAF JUICE	Has great benefits in skin protection and repair; its soothing, cooling and healing effects are well documented.
ARGAN OIL ◌ @	ARGANIA SPINOSA KERNEL OIL	Has been used for centuries by Berber women in Morocco to nourish their skin, hair and nails. It is exceptionally rich in natural tocopherols, carotenes, squalene and essential fatty acids.
ASTRAGALUS (FROM CAPSULE) ◌ @	ASTRAGALUS MEMBRANACEUS	Very effective against glycation, which reduces the ability of collagen fibre in the skin to regenerate, leading to the wrinkling and sagging that characterize skin-ageing.

COMMON NAME	INCI (EU) NAME	BENEFIT
AVOCADO OIL ☺🗑	PERSEA GRATISSIMA OIL	Obtained by pressing the dehydrated, sliced flesh of the avocado pear. Consisting primarily of the glycerides of linoleic, oleic and palmitic fatty acids, it improves moisturization and softens rough, dry skin.
BANANA FOOD FLAVOUR 🗑	NATURAL FLAVOURING, PROPYLENE GLYCOL	Natural banana flavour for lip balms.
BASIL ESSENTIAL OIL ☺@	OCIMUM BASILICUM HERB OIL	An aromatic oil that contributes to the fragrance of the product and is reputed to help stimulate the scalp and promote hair growth; also effective against acne.
BEER 🗑	BEER	The nutrient proteins and B vitamins found in beer help to nourish and strengthen dry, damaged hair, adding manageability and shine.
BEESWAX WHITE BP ☺@	CERA ALBA	The wax obtained from the honeycomb formed by the bee. It forms a protective barrier on the surface of the skin that provides a shield against irritants, while still allowing the skin to breathe.
BLADDERWRACK SEAWEED, GROUND @	FUCUS VESICULOSUS	A rich source of beta-carotene, antioxidants, iodine, bromine, potassium and many other minerals, as well as skin-replenishing polysaccharides; is reputed to be beneficial against cellulite and have anti-ageing properties.
BORAGE (STARFLOWER) OIL ☺@	BORAGO OFFICINALIS SEED OIL	Rich in omega-3 and omega-6 essential fatty acids, which help to restore the skin's barrier function and reduce trans-epidermal water loss; also improves skin elasticity and firmness, and is ideal for dry, itchy skin.
CALENDULA (MARIGOLD) PETALS @	CALENDULA OFFICINALIS	Best known for its antimicrobial and anti-inflammatory properties; helps to soothe burns, insect bites, eczema, skin ulcers and rashes.

COMMON NAME	INCI (EU) NAME	BENEFIT
CAMOMILE ESSENTIAL OIL ○@	ANTHEMIS NOBILIS OIL	English or Roman camomile oil is an aromatic oil that contributes to the fragrance of the product and, owing to the active content of bisabolol, has effective skin-soothing properties.
CAMOMILE INFUSION ○@	CHAMOMILLA RECUTITA FLOWER EXTRACT	See Camomile tea.
CAMOMILE TEA ○🧺	CHAMOMILLA RECUTITA FLOWER EXTRACT	Renowned for its many skincare benefits, including skin soothing and calming, plus radiance and brightening.
CARAMEL FOOD FLAVOUR 🧺	GLYCERINE, WATER, PROPYLENE GLYCOL, NATURAL FLAVOURING, COLOUR: PLAIN CARAMEL	Natural caramel flavour for lip balms.
CETEARYL ALCOHOL @	CETEARYL ALCOHOL	A thickener and co-emulsifier for creams and lotions, derived from plant origin.
CHIA SEEDS ○@🧺	SALVIA HISPANICA SEEDS	The seeds from this Mexican flowering plant have a high oil content that is rich in omega-3 fatty acids, making them an ideal soft scrub agent for dry and sensitive skins.
CHLORELLA (TABLET) ○@	CHLORELLA VULGARIS EXTRACT	This extract of green microalgae is shown to firm, strengthen and tone the skin by increasing collagen and elastin production; also helps to regulate microcirculation, thus reducing the appearance of fine blood vessels.
CIDER VINEGAR ○🧺	PYRUS MALUS FRUIT EXTRACT	Helps to maintain the pH balance of hair and removes product build-up without stripping hair of its natural oils; seals down the cuticles, resulting in smoother, softer and shinier hair. It also has antimicrobial properties and can help to prevent dandruff.
CINNAMON LEAF ESSENTIAL OIL ○@	CINNAMOMUM CULILAWAN LEAF OIL	A warm, spicy oil renowned for its distinctive aroma and antimicrobial properties.

COMMON NAME	INCI (EU) NAME	BENEFIT
CITRIC ACID ✛@	CITRIC ACID	A pH modifier.
COCOA BUTTER @	THEOBROMA CACAO SEED BUTTER	A creamy butter that melts at body temperature and is renowned for its excellent emollient properties; soothes, softens and protects the skin.
COCONUT MILK ⌓🧺	COCOS NUCIFERA FRUIT JUICE	Derived from the flesh of the coconut; can be used for cleansing the skin, to impart a soft, supple and radiant complexion. It also helps to keep the skin hydrated and moisturized.
COCONUT OIL, UNREFINED ⌓🧺	COCOS NUCIFERA OIL	Rich in fatty acids, triglycerides and natural tocopherol; has excellent protective and moisturizing properties, and can be used on both skin and hair.
COCONUT WATER ⌓🧺	COCOS NUCIFERA WATER	Called *noelani*, meaning 'dew from the heavens', by the Hawaiians; helps to refresh and hydrate the skin.
COENZYME Q10 (TABLET) ✛⌓@	UBIQUINONE	Helps to boost skin repair and regeneration, and reduces free-radical damage.
CORNFLOUR (CORNSTARCH) 🧺	ZEA MAYS	A fine powder often used as a natural thickener or a cosmetic powder base that imparts a smooth feel to the skin.
CUCUMBER 🧺	CUCUMIS SATIVUS FRUIT EXTRACT	Renowned for its skin-cooling and soothing effects.
CYPRESS ESSENTIAL OIL ⌓@	CUPRESSUS SEMPERVIRENS OIL	An aromatic oil extracted from the small branches and leaves of the tree through steam distillation. A venous decongestant and vasoconstrictor, it has healing properties, particularly in the case of varicose veins.
DISTILLED WITCH HAZEL BPC ✛	ALCOHOL DENAT. (and) HAMAMELIS VIRGINIANA BARK/LEAF/TWIG EXTRACT	A renowned natural astringent, skin toner and skin refresher.

COMMON NAME	INCI (EU) NAME	BENEFIT
DRIED MILK POWDER 🧺	WHOLE DRY MILK	The natural fats in whole milk powder help to moisturize and soften the skin.
ELDERFLOWER @	SAMBUCUS NIGRA	Used to soften the skin and to treat acne, blemishes, rashes and sunburn; also reputed to help fade freckles and reduce wrinkles.
ELDERFLOWER INFUSION @	SAMBUCUS NIGRA EXTRACT	See Elderflower.
EMULSIFYING WAX BP @	CETEARYL ALCOHOL (and) SODIUM LAURYL SULFATE	A general-purpose emulsifier that enables oil and water to combine easily to form a stable cream.
EPSOM SALTS ✚ 🍎	MAGNESIUM SULFATE	A mineral easily absorbed by the skin; helps to soothe and relax the body, relieve aches and ease muscular pains.
ESP ORGANIC SAFEMULS SCA @	ALOE BARBADENSIS LEAF JUICE (and) SUCROSE COCOATE	A combination of aloe vera extract and a natural emulsifier derived from coconut oil and sugar; has exceptional skin-softening properties. It enables oil and water to combine easily to form a stable cream.
EUCALYPTUS ESSENTIAL OIL 🍎 @	EUCALYPTUS GLOBULUS LEAF OIL	An aromatic oil obtained from the leaves of the tree; has anti-inflammatory, antimicrobial and stimulating properties.
EVENING PRIMROSE OIL ✚ 🍎	OENOTHERA BIENNIS OIL	Rich in essential fatty acids and gamma linoleic acid, which help to maintain the moisture barrier of the skin; helps to soothe and protect dry skin.
FENNEL ESSENTIAL OIL 🍎 @	FOENICULUM VULGARE OIL	An aromatic oil distilled from the seeds of the plant; has antimicrobial properties and is also helpful against cellulite.
FRACTIONATED COCONUT OIL 🍎	CAPRYLIC/CAPRIC TRIGLYCERIDE	A fine emollient, extracted from coconut oil, that leaves a light but silky-skin feel without greasiness.

COMMON NAME	INCI (EU) NAME	BENEFIT
FRANKINCENSE ESSENTIAL OIL ⏧@	BOSWELLIA CARTERII OIL	Frankincense, also known as olibanum, is extracted from the tree resin and is known for its anti-ageing and skin-toning properties.
GERANIUM ESSENTIAL OIL ⏧@	PELARGONIUM GRAVEOLENS FLOWER OIL	The characteristic floral odour of this oil makes it ideal for skincare fragrancing. It also has antimicrobial and astringent properties, making it beneficial for natural deodorants.
GINSENG (FROM CAPSULE) ✚⏧@	PANAX GINSENG	Contains a large amount of phytonutrients, which can stimulate and activate the skin's metabolism, and are thus ideal for anti-ageing treatments.
GLYCERINE ✚🗑	GLYCERIN	A highly effective humectant, derived from palm oil, that helps to maintain the moisture balance and hydrate parched skin; one of the oldest and most respected skin moisturizers.
GOTU KOLA (TABLET) ⏧@	CENTELLA ASIATICA LEAF EXTRACT	The active components of this plant stimulate the renewal of collagen to help strengthen vascular walls and restore elasticity to improve firmness and skin tone.
GRAPEFRUIT ESSENTIAL OIL ⏧@	CITRUS GRANDIS PEEL OIL	A zesty, refreshing aromatic oil extracted from the fruit peel; has excellent cleansing properties and is ideal for oily skin.
GRAPEFRUIT SEED EXTRACT ⏧@	CITRUS GRANDIS SEED EXTRACT	See Preservative GSE.
GRAPESEED OIL ⏧🗑	VITIS VINIFERA SEED OIL	Has a very light feel on the skin, is easily absorbed and helps to reduce water loss.
GREEN CLAY @	ILLITE	Has long been known for its detoxifying skincare benefits, which can be attributed to its unique mineral composition; helps to absorb skin impurities and is mostly recommended for oily, clogged or acneic skin.

COMMON NAME	INCI (EU) NAME	BENEFIT
GREEN TEA ☌🧺	CAMELLIA SINENSIS	Contains polyphenols, which have antioxidant and anti-inflammatory activities that can offer anti-ageing properties and help to protect the skin against damage caused by free radicals.
GREEN TEA INFUSION ☌🧺	CAMELLIA SINENSIS LEAF EXTRACT	See Green tea.
GROUND PUMICE @	PUMICE	These hard grains of volcanic rock make an ideal exfoliant for removing hard skin from tired feet.
IVY INFUSION @	HEDERA HELIX EXTRACT	The leaf extract of this climbing plant is well known for its antimicrobial and anti-cellulite properties.
JASMINE ESSENTIAL OIL ☌@	JASMINUM OFFICINALE OIL	An exotic aromatic oil extracted from the flowers of the plant. It has a strongly sweet, uplifting fragrance that is very common in flowers that bloom only at night; also has antimicrobial properties, but is generally used for its fragrance.
JOJOBA OIL ☌	SIMMONDSIA CHINENSIS SEED OIL	A highly penetrating, rich oil that closely resembles natural sebum; can be used to help balance the skin's natural oils, and also contains natural antioxidants.
JUNIPER ESSENTIAL OIL ☌@	JUNIPERUS COMMUNIS FRUIT OIL	An aromatic oil obtained from the needles, wood and fruit of the shrub; has excellent antimicrobial and astringent properties.
KAOLIN (WHITE CLAY) ☌@	KAOLIN	A soft white clay, commonly referred to as 'China clay' (on account of the hill, Kao-ling, in China from which it was mined for centuries), that helps to draw impurities and toxins from the skin.
LAGER 🧺	BEER	See Beer.

COMMON NAME	INCI (EU) NAME	BENEFIT
LAMESOFT PO 65 @	AQUA (and) CITRIC ACID (and) COCO-GLUCOSIDE (and) GLYCERYL OLEATE (and) HYDROGENATED PALM GLYCERIDES CITRATE (and) TOCOPHEROL	Naturally derived from coconut oil and sunflower oil, this additive in surfactant/foaming cleansers has positive moisturizing effects on the skin.
LAVENDER ESSENTIAL OIL ✚⏲@	LAVANDULA ANGUSTIFOLIA OIL	An aromatic oil with many skincare benefits on account of its soothing and antimicrobial properties; renowned for its relaxing fragrance, it is ideal for night-time.
LAVENDER FLOWERS @	LAVANDULA ANGUSTIFOLIA	In Roman times the flowers were added to baths, hence the name; the Latin verb *lavare* means 'to wash'. The fragrant dried flowers give a pleasing visual texture and delicate fragrance to bath powders and body scrubs.
LEAF GELATINE 🛒	PORK GELATIN	Largely composed of the amino acids glycine and proline, which are required for proper skin, hair and nail growth and are anti-inflammatory; may also help to speed the healing of wounds.
LEMON ESSENTIAL OIL ⏲@	CITRUS LIMON PEEL OIL	A fresh citrus aromatic oil that helps to brighten and rejuvenate sagging or tired-looking skin; also recommended for reducing excessive oil on the skin. Its antimicrobial properties help to treat skin disorders such as acne. Effective as a hair tonic to help promote strong, healthy and shiny hair and to eliminate dandruff.
LEMON JUICE 🛒	CITRUS LIMON JUICE	A natural source of the non-abrasive exfoliant AHA citric acid; ideal for oily skin and also has skin-brightening properties.
LEMON ZEST 🛒	CITRUS MEDICA LIMONUM PEEL POWDER	The ground, dried peel of lemon is ideal as a soft exfoliator in hand and body scrubs.
LEMONGRASS ESSENTIAL OIL ⏲@	CYMBOPOGON SCHOENANTHUS OIL	A lemony aromatic oil that contributes to the fragrance of the product and has a mild deodorizing effect.

COMMON NAME	INCI (EU) NAME	BENEFIT
LIME ESSENTIAL OIL ○@	CITRUS AURANTIFOLIA OIL	An aromatic citrus peel oil with antimicrobial properties that helps to fight acne and dandruff.
LINSEED (FLAXSEED) ○🧺	LINUM USITATISSIMUM	The seeds of the flax plant are high in nourishing omega-3 fatty acids. When they are boiled in water, the resulting gel is perfect for hair styling, leaving it soft, shiny, moisturized and with great curl definition.
LIQUORICE INFUSION ○	GLYCYRRHIZA GLABRA ROOT EXTRACT	Helps to even out tone and add radiance to the skin.
MACADAMIA NUT OIL ○	MACADAMIA TERNIFOLIA SEED OIL	Contains the highest level in any plant oil of palmitoleic acid, which is found in youthful skin, but the level of which reduces in mature skin. Also rich in calming and healing phytosterols, making it a perfect oil for repairing the skin's barrier function.
MANUKA HONEY ○🧺	MEL	Ideal for blemished skin because of its natural antibacterial and anti-inflammatory properties; also helps to balance the skin's pH and is a natural humectant, helping the skin to retain moisture.
MINT WATER @	MENTHA PIPERITA LEAF WATER	A natural toner that helps to keep the skin oil-free and fresh; also helps to even skin tone and reduce puffiness around the eyes.
NATURAL PINK FOOD COLOURING 🧺	PROPYLENE GLYCOL, COLOUR BEETROOT RED, WATER, ANTIOXIDANT, ASCORBIC ACID, PRESERVATIVE POTASSIUM SORBATE	Food colourant based on beetroot, used for lip and cheek tint.
NEROLI ESSENTIAL OIL ○@	CITRUS AURANTIUM AMARA OIL	An uplifting aromatic oil made from orange flowers; can be used as a body perfume and, due to its potent antimicrobial properties, is also beneficial for skincare.
OAT BRAN ○	AVENA SATIVA	See Porridge oats.

COMMON NAME	INCI (EU) NAME	BENEFIT
OAT FLOUR ○	AVENA SATIVA	A fine powder of ground oats that helps to smooth and exfoliate the skin; also absorbs and removes excess oil and bacteria, thus helping to combat acne.
OLIVE OIL ⏇	OLEA EUROPAEA FRUIT OIL	Obtained from the ripe fruit of the olive tree. Consisting primarily of the glycerides of linoleic, oleic and palmitic fatty acids, it is reputed to help skin-cell regeneration.
OLIVEM 1000 @	CETEARYL OLIVATE (and) SORBITAN OLIVATE	A natural emulsifier derived from olive oil. It is easy to use and also has skin-moisturizing benefits.
ORANGE ESSENTIAL OIL, SWEET ○@	CITRUS AURANTIUM DULCIS PEEL OIL	An aromatic oil, obtained from orange peel, that creates a happy, uplifted mood; also has antimicrobial and cleansing properties and helps to brighten the skin.
ORANGE FLOWER WATER @⏇	CITRUS AURANTIUM AMARA FLOWER DISTILLATE	A delicately fragrant water, produced from the distillation of orange flower petals, that helps to soothe and refresh the skin.
ORANGE ZEST ⏇	CITRUS AURANTIUM DULCIS PEEL POWDER	The ground, dried peel of orange is ideal as a soft exfoliator in hand and body scrubs.
PAPAYA ENZYME (TABLET) ○@	CARICA PAPAYA FRUIT EXTRACT	Contains several unique proteolytic enzymes, including papain, that help to renew the complexion by dissolving dead skin cells and accelerating cell renewal.
PEPPERMINT ESSENTIAL OIL ○@	MENTHA PIPERITA OIL	An aromatic oil containing menthol, which creates a cooling sensation to refresh tired skin; also beneficial for oily skin. It is excellent for rejuvenating the hair follicles, stimulating the scalp and promoting hair growth.

COMMON NAME	INCI (EU) NAME	BENEFIT
PETITGRAIN ESSENTIAL OIL ⏱@	CITRUS AURANTIUM AMARA LEAF/ TWIG OIL	A popular perfumery ingredient with an uplifting aroma, extracted from the fresh leaves and young and tender twigs of the orange tree through steam distillation. Has deodorizing and antimicrobial properties, making it useful for treating skin infections.
PINE ESSENTIAL OIL ⏱@	PINUS SYLVESTRIS TWIG LEAF OIL	An aromatic oil that helps to reduce inflammation and associated redness, especially in skin conditions such as eczema and psoriasis; also has antioxidant properties and helps to mop up free radicals that can lead to premature ageing of the skin.
PINEAPPLE 🧺	ANANAS SATIVUS	Contains bromelain, which is an enzyme that naturally exfoliates the skin by effectively 'dissolving' dead skin cells, leaving the skin feeling clean and soft.
PINK CLAY @	KAOLIN	French pink clay (Argiletz clay) is a gentle combination of red and white clays that can be used to cleanse and detoxify normal to dry skin, remove dead skin cells and create a refreshed appearance.
PLANTAPON LGC @	SODIUM LAURYL GLUCOSE CARBOXYLATE (and) LAURYL GLUCOSIDE	A mild cleansing and foaming base derived from natural coconut oil and sugar origins. It is ideal for shower gels, shampoos and facial cleansers.
POLYSORBATE 20 @	POLYSORBATE 20	A natural solubilizer, derived from sugar, that enables essential oils, oils and fragrance to mix in with an aqueous base.
PORRIDGE OATS ⏱🧺	AVENA SATIVA	Contains beta-glucan, which forms a fine protective film and penetrates the skin to provide deep moisturization. Also has anti-inflammatory properties that are effective in healing dry and itchy skin.

COMMON NAME	INCI (EU) NAME	BENEFIT
PRESERVATIVE GSE (GRAPEFRUIT SEED EXTRACT) ☺@	CITRUS GRANDIS SEED EXTRACT	A bioflavonoid concentrate prepared from the seeds, pulp and white membranes of grapefruit, used as a broad-spectrum, non-toxic antimicrobial compound.
RED FOOD COLOURING 🗑	WATER, COLOURS, ANTHOCYANIN, PAPRIKA EXTRACT, CITRIC ACID, PROPYLENE GLYCOL, EMULSIFIER, POLYOXYETHYLENE, SORBITAN MONOOLEATE	Food colourant based on paprika, used for lip and cheek tint.
RESVERATROL (FROM CAPSULE) ☺@	COMPLEX BLEND WITH RESVERATROL	A potent antioxidant found in foods such as grapes, some berries and red wine. When applied topically, it protects the skin against sun damage, improves collagen synthesis and reduces cell damage, so is an effective anti-ageing ingredient.
RHODIOLA (FROM CAPSULE) ☺@	RHODIOLA ROSEA ROOT EXTRACT	The plant, also known as golden root or rose root, grows in mountainous parts of Europe and other cold regions of the world. The root extract stimulates lipolysis (fat-burning) and is shown to actively reduce under-eye puffiness by driving lipolysis at the cellular level.
RICE BRAN ☺	ORYZA SATIVA	A soft and nourishing exfoliator, ideal for dry, troubled skin.
RICE BRAN OIL ☺ 🗑	ORYZA SATIVA BRAN OIL	An excellent natural, non-greasy emollient and moisturizer. Rich in antioxidant vitamin E and gamma-oryzanol, it protects against free radicals and skin dryness.
ROSE WATER ☺ 🗑	ROSA DAMASCENA FLOWER WATER	Adds a delicate fragrance to the product and is also reputed to be soothing and toning.

COMMON NAME	INCI (EU) NAME	BENEFIT
ROSEHIP OIL ⏱@	ROSA CANINA FRUIT OIL	Rich in omega-3, omega-6, vitamin A and antioxidant tocopherols; helps to protect, repair and restore the skin and maintain its moisture balance.
ROSEMARY ESSENTIAL OIL ✛⏱@	ROSMARINUS OFFICINALIS LEAF OIL	Regular use of this aromatic oil helps to stimulate hair follicles, nourishes the scalp and removes dandruff; also believed to slow down premature hair loss and greying of the hair. Has antimicrobial properties and can help to tone the skin.
ROSEMARY INFUSION 🧺	ROSMARINUS OFFICINALIS EXTRACT	See Rosemary leaves.
ROSEMARY LEAVES 🧺	ROSMARINUS OFFICINALIS	Contains polyphenols and rosmarinic acid, and is reputed to have antioxidant and antimicrobial properties.
SAGE INFUSION 🧺	SALVIA OFFICINALIS LEAF EXTRACT	A great toner for regulating sebum production in oily complexions; has antimicrobial and anti-inflammatory properties, which help against acne, as well as relieve symptoms of troubled dry skin. Also helps to stimulate hair growth.
SEA SALT, COARSE OR FINE ⏱🧺	MARIS SAL	A complex blend of minerals and trace elements that optimize cell performance; it is detoxifying and also acts as an exfoliator to remove dead skin cells and leave the skin clean, smooth and soft.
SEAWEED INFUSION (SERRATED WRACK) @	FUCUS SERRATUS EXTRACT	An olive-brown shrubby seaweed containing natural antioxidant compounds that have long been known to have pronounced anti-ageing, skin-conditioning, repair and hydrating effects.
SHEA BUTTER @	BUTYROSPERMUM PARKII BUTTER	Has a unique fatty acid profile such that it readily melts at body temperature, making it an ideal emollient for skin; also has soothing and protective properties.

COMMON NAME	INCI (EU) NAME	BENEFIT
SODIUM BICARBONATE (BAKING SODA) 👐 🧺	SODIUM BICARBONATE	The natural mineral form of sodium bicarbonate is nahcolite, often found dissolved in mineral springs. It can be used in natural cosmetics as a deodorant and to clean and smooth the skin. Sodium bicarbonate generates the 'fizz' in bath bombs when it is combined with citric acid in the presence of water.
SOLUBLE ASPIRIN (TABLET) ✚	ACETYLSALICYLIC ACID	Contains acetylsalicylic and a small amount of salicylic acid; can help to soothe and brighten the skin.
SPARKLING WATER 🧺	AQUA	A natural source of hydrating water containing minerals and trace elements, as well as carbon dioxide gas to add a refreshing fizz.
SPEARMINT ESSENTIAL OIL 👐 @	MENTHA SPICATA HERB OIL	An aromatic oil extracted from the flowering tops of the spearmint plant through steam distillation. It does not contain as much menthol as peppermint and, as such, is not as cooling, but does have antimicrobial properties.
SPRING WATER 🧺	AQUA	A natural source of water containing minerals and trace elements to help rehydrate the skin.
SUCRAGEL CF @	AQUA (and) CAPRYLIC/CAPRIC TRIGLYCERIDE (and) GLYCERIN (and) SUCROSE LAURATE	A natural emulsifier blend derived from plant sugars and coconut palm oils. It is gentle on the skin and leaves it with an ultra-soft conditioned feel.
SWEET ALMOND OIL 👐	PRUNUS AMYGDALUS DULCIS OIL	Naturally rich in essential fatty acids and vitamins A, B1, B2, B6 and E; an excellent emollient for softening the skin.
TANGERINE ESSENTIAL OIL 👐 @	CITRUS RETICULATA PEEL OIL	A fresh citrus aromatic oil extracted by cold compression of tangerine peel; improves circulation and helps to maintain oil and moisture balance in the skin.

COMMON NAME	INCI (EU) NAME	BENEFIT
TEA TREE ESSENTIAL OIL ✚ ⭕ @	MELALEUCA ALTERNIFOLIA OIL	A traditional remedy originally used by the Aboriginal Australians to treat bruises, insect bites and skin infections; has very effective antimicrobial properties.
THYME ESSENTIAL OIL ⭕ @	THYMUS VULGARIS OIL	An aromatic oil extracted from the fresh flowers and leaves of the plant through steam distillation; has medicinal and antimicrobial properties, and is effective against insect stings and bites.
THYME INFUSION ⬜	THYMUS VULGARIS EXTRACT	Has antimicrobial properties and can help to control acne.
TIN OXIDE @	TIN OXIDE	An ultra-fine abrasive powder used to buff nails and give them a high shine.
UNPERFUMED SOAP ✚ ⭕	SODIUM STEARATE, SODIUM COCOATE, SODIUM PALMITATE (may vary)	Soaps are made from fats and oils that react with lye (sodium hydroxide). Solid fats such as coconut oil and palm oil are used to ensure the soap stays hard and does not dissolve in the water left in the soap dish. Soaps have a high pH; they are used for skin cleansing and are effective at dispersing oil and grease.
VITAMIN C ✚ ⭕ @	ASCORBIC ACID	Pure vitamin C is renowned for its potent antioxidant properties. It helps to brighten the skin, reduces the appearance of age spots and other types of sun damage, and also boosts healthy collagen production.
VITAMIN E ✚ ⭕ @	TOCOPHEROL	Found widely throughout nature, particularly in wheatgerm oil. It is an effective antioxidant and free-radical scavenger, and so helps to protect the skin from environmental damage; has also been found to be beneficial in scar reduction and wound-healing.

COMMON NAME	INCI (EU) NAME	BENEFIT
VODKA	ALCOHOL	A carrier and solvent for essential oils.
WHEATGERM OIL	TRITICUM VULGARE GERM OIL	Readily absorbed by the skin, delivering an infusion of vitamins, antioxidants, fatty acids and phytosterols, which help to moisturize and heal dry or cracked skin, and also prevent scarring; in particular, a rich source of vitamin E, which helps to reduce skin damage, fight free radicals, support healthy collagen formation and maintain even skin tone.
WHITE CLAY	KAOLIN	See Kaolin.
XANTHAN GUM	XANTHAN GUM	A thickener/stabilizer naturally derived from corn sugar through a biofermentation process; commonly used in foods.
YARROW INFUSION	ACHILLEA MILLEFOLIUM EXTRACT	Has astringent and anti-inflammatory properties, and is beneficial for dry and troubled skin.
YLANG-YLANG ESSENTIAL OIL	CANANGA ODORATA FLOWER OIL	An uplifting aromatic oil extracted from the fresh flowers of the ylang-ylang tree through steam distillation; mostly used for its exotic fragrance, but can help to maintain moisture and oil balance, keeping the skin looking hydrated and smooth.
YOGHURT	YOGURT	Contains zinc and lactic acid, which promote healthy skin; also helps to remove dead skin cells, smooth fine lines, tighten pores, hydrate dry patches and leave the skin radiant.

Directory of Suppliers

UK

ABSOLUTE AROMAS
absolute-aromas.com
Specialist online supplier of essential oils, with an extensive selection; also sells carrier oils.
Ships internationally.

AMPULLA
ampulla.co.uk
Online packaging supplier, selling glass, plastic and aluminium containers for cosmetics and food. Offers an excellent selection, with pricing from a single item to bulk quantities.
Also has a European site: ampulla.eu

AROMANTIC
aromantic.co.uk
Online supplier of cosmetic ingredients, containers and kits. Also offers skincare and cosmetic courses in Scotland (where the company is based) and London.
Ships internationally.

G. BALDWIN & CO.
baldwins.co.uk
171/173 Walworth Road, London SE17 1RW
Retail store and online supplier of herbs, as well as vitamins and supplements. Also offers skincare courses in London.
Ships internationally.

BATH POTTERS' SUPPLIES
bathpotters.co.uk
Supplier of pottery materials, including tin oxide, used in our Nail Buffer recipe.

COMPAK SOUTH
compaksouth.com
Online supplier of glass packaging. Specializes in food containers, but also sells lever-top jars, small bottles and jars, and closures for cosmetics, as well as a few plastic items.

EASY FLORIST SUPPLIES
easyfloristsupplies.co.uk
Online supplier of gift bags and cellophane (suitable for wrapping bath bombs), as well as tissue paper and kraft papers.

GRACEFRUIT
gracefruit.com
Online supplier of cosmetic ingredients. Also sells packaging, fragrances and flavours, and bases.
Ships to Europe.

HOLLAND AND BARRETT
hollandandbarrett.com
Large chain of health-food stores, located in most medium-sized/large towns in the UK. Sells food ingredients, including nuts, seeds and cereals, as well as vitamins, supplements and essential oils.

THE SOAP KITCHEN
thesoapkitchen.co.uk
The Soap Kitchen Plus, 11a South Street
Torrington, Devon EX38 8AA
Retail store and online supplier of a wide range of cosmetic ingredients, starter kits and bath bomb and soap moulds. Also offers courses in making soap, creams and bath bombs, as well as technical advice.
Has pricing in euros, and ships to Europe.

USA

BRAMBLE BERRY
brambleberry.com
Online supplier of soap-making and other cosmetic ingredients, essential oils, moulds and packaging. Offers courses in soap-making.
Ships internationally.

THE CHEMISTRY STORE

chemistrystore.com

Online supplier of soap-making and other cosmetic ingredients, equipment and packaging.
Ships internationally.

FROM NATURE WITH LOVE

fromnaturewithlove.com

Online supplier of cosmetic ingredients, equipment, packaging and books.
Ships internationally.

THE HERBARIE

theherbarie.com

Online supplier of cosmetic ingredients, packaging and books.
Ships to North America.

MAKING COSMETICS

makingcosmetics.com

Online supplier of cosmetic ingredients, vitamins, fragrances, equipment, packaging and books.
Ships internationally.

AUSTRALIA AND NEW ZEALAND

AUSSIE SOAP SUPPLIES

aussiesoapsupplies.com.au

Online supplier of ingredients for soap-making, cosmetics and skincare, including floral waters, botanicals and kits.
Ships to selected countries.

ESCENTIALS OF AUSTRALIA

escentialsofaustralia.com

Online supplier of ingredients for soap-making, cosmetics, essential oils, skin- and haircare products, and packaging.
Ships internationally.

NEW DIRECTIONS

newdirections.com.au

Online supplier of essential oils, herbal extracts, cosmetic ingredients, cosmeceuticals, equipment and packaging; also sells Australian specialities, listed as native botanical skincare.
Ships internationally.

SOAP NATURALLY/SOAP NATCH

soapnaturally.org

Online resource for those interested in soap-making and handmade skincare, with information on suppliers and classes and workshops in Australia and New Zealand.

EUROPE

AROMA ZONE

aroma-zone.com

French online supplier of cosmetic ingredients, natural extracts and essential oils, as well as packaging.

DRAGONSPICE

dragonspice.de

German online health-food supplier with some cosmetic ingredients.

JABONARIUM

jabonariumshop.com

Spanish online supplier of cosmetic ingredients, essential oils, fragrances and packaging.

MANSKE

manske-shop.com

German online supplier of cosmetic ingredients, essential oils, equipment and packaging.

Index

Acknowledgements

We would like to thank the team at Jacqui Small for commissioning this book. Particular thanks go to our ever-vigilant editor, Claire Chandler, for her incredible eye for detail, and also to Rachel Cross, Amanda Heywood and Sophie Martell, for making the projects really come to life on the page.

Juliette: I would like to thank the many volunteer testers, both at the classes and among our friends and families, who gave us their helpful comments. But my special thanks go to my daughter Caitlin, my favourite beauty-product critic and fan, and of course to Abi, for sharing her incredible knowledge.

Abi: I would like to thank Juliette for inviting me to co-write this book and for her boundless enthusiasm in trialling all the recipes. Thanks also to Ozzie, for sitting at my feet for hours on end, instead of going for his walk.

About the Authors

Juliette Goggin runs a consulting company specializing in product development for skincare, toiletries and home fragrance. She has worked with many niche brands to create innovative new products, and is a regular speaker at cosmetic industry seminars. She initially trained in the fragrance industry, and later went on to create her own range of candles and soaps. Juliette runs crafting classes from her home in East Sussex, teaching home-made skincare, candle-making and jewellery design. She appeared in two series of *SuperScrimpers* on Channel 4, and is the co-author of *Junk Genius*, published in 2012.

Abi Righton is a respected cosmetic scientist. She has almost 40 years' experience in formulating beauty and personal care products, including for the Body Shop, and she now runs her own business offering cosmetic formulations based on natural ingredients and new technologies. Her services are sought by premium skincare, haircare and spa brands worldwide.

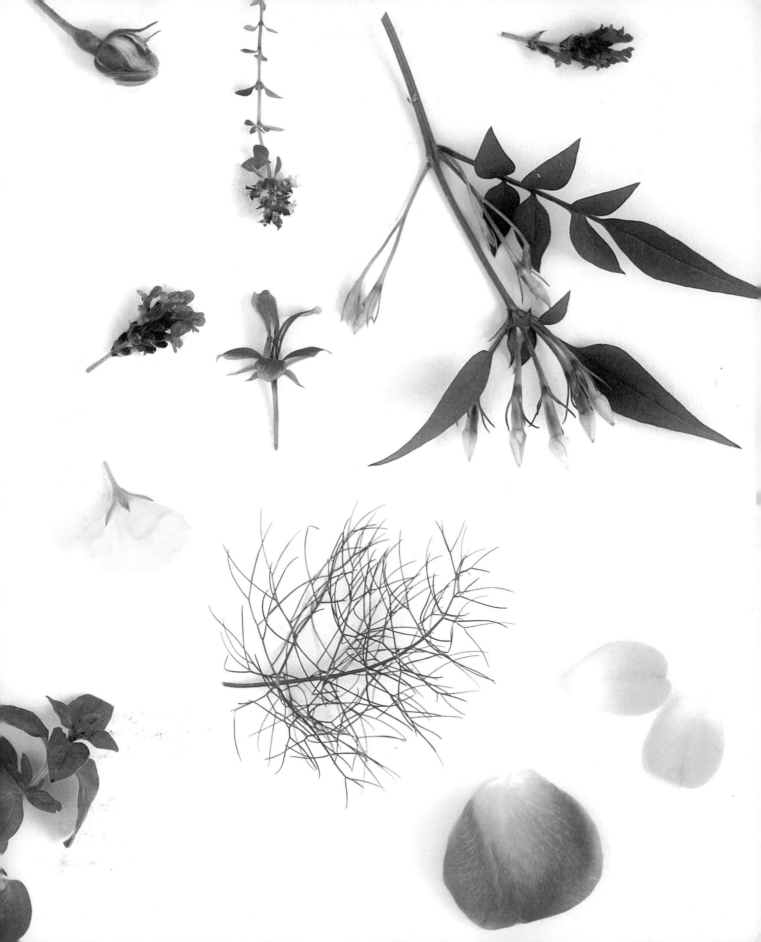